Interfaces in Total Hip Arthı

Springer-Verlag London Ltd.

Ian D. Learmonth (Ed)

Interfaces in Total Hip Arthroplasty

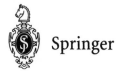 Springer

Ian D. Learmonth, MB, ChB, FRCS, FRCS Ed, FCS (SA) Orth
Professor and Head, Department of Orthopaedic Surgery, University of Bristol
Honorary Consultant, Bristol Royal Infirmary and Southmead Hospital

ISBN 978-1-4471-1150-4

British Library Cataloguing in Publication Data
Interfaces in total hip arthroplasty
  1. Total hip replacement
  I. Learmonth, Ian D.
  617.5'81'0592
  ISBN 978-1-4471-1150-4

Library of Congress Cataloging-in-Publication Data
Interfaces in total hip arthroplasty / Ian D. Learmonth (ed.)
    p. cm.
  Includes bibliographical references and index.
  ISBN 978-1-4471-1150-4   ISBN 978-1-4471-0477-3 (eBook)
  DOI 10.1007/978-1-4471-0477-3
  1. Artifical hip joints. 2. Biomedical materials. 3. Biological interfaces.
  4. Total hip replacement. I. Learmonth, Ian D., 1945- .
  [DNLM: 1. Arthroplasty, Replacement, Hip. 2. Biocompatible Materials.   WE 860 I59 1999]
RD549.I57   1999
617.5'810592—dc21
DNLM/DLC
for Library of Congress   99–40676

© Springer-Verlag London 2000
Originally published by Springer-Verlag London Berlin Hiedelberg in 2000
Softcover reprint of the hardcover 1st edition 2000

Typeset by Florence Production Ld, Stoodleigh, Devon, England

28/3830-543210 Printed on acid-free paper SPIN 10672011

Preface

This book incorporates the experience of numerous experts who explore contemporary opinion of how best to rationalise and optimise the interfaces at total hip replacement to provide the most favourable and durable results.

The survival of a total hip replacement depends principally on the enduring integrity of the fixation interfaces and of the articular interface. The design of the stem and the material properties of cement largely determine the state of the component-cement interface, while the bone-cement interface is significantly influenced by both mechanical and biological factors. The surface finish and shape of cementless implants are designed to preserve the integrity of biological fixation (osseo-integration) at the bone-component interface. Once again, both mechanical and biological factors have to be considered, while bioactive coatings accelerate bone ongrowth.

Metal-on-polyethylene is the most widely used articular interface. However, it has been suggested that wear of polyethylene is one of the major factors contributing to failure of total hip replacements. The increasing prevalence of total hip replacement in younger patients has stimulated the investigation of alternative, more durable couples – including ceramic-polyethylene, ceramic-ceramic and metal-on-metal.

Modularity provides greater intra-operative flexibility, but each new modular interface introduces new mechanisms of failure. These need to be anticipated and appropriate measures taken to avoid them.

Hopefully this book will provide a better understanding of the factors that contribute to stable interfaces and long-term survival of total hip arthroplasty.

I.D. Learmonth

Acknowledgements

This book is based on the proceedings of a symposium on Interfaces in Total Hip Arthroplasty held at the Aesculapium in Tuttlingen under the auspices of Aesculap Academia.

Mrs Martha van der Lem is to be thanked for her and editorial assistance and general support.

Contents

Contributors

Mr A.A. Besong
Research Student
Medical and Biological Engineering Group
Department of Microbiology
University of Leeds, Leeds LS2 9JT, UK

Prof. Dr. med. A. Braun
Vulpius Klinik GmbH
Abteilung Orthopadie
Vulpiusstraße 29
D-74899 Bad Rappenau, Germany

Dipl.-Ing. G.H. Buchhorn
Biomaterial Laboratory
Orthopaedic Hospital
University of Göttingen
Robert-Koch-Straße 40
D-37075 Gottingen, Germany

Mr G.J. Charnley
Derriford Hospital
Derriford Road
Plymouth PL6 8DH, UK

Mr J.D.J. Eldridge
Department of Orthopaedic Surgery
Level 5
Bristol Royal Infirmary
Bristol BS2 8HW, UK

Professor J. Fisher
Professor of Mechanical Engineering
Medical and Biological Engineering Group
Department of Mechanical Engineering
University of Leeds, Leeds LS2 9JT, UK

Dr L. Frommelt
Head of Department
Bacterio-Serological Laboratory
ENDO-KLINIK
Holstenstraße 2
D-22767 Hamburg, Germany

Dr C. Garreau de Loubresse
Service Chirurgie Général II
Traumatologie et Orthopedie
Hôpital Tenon, 4 rue de la Chine
75970 Paris Cedex 20, France

Dr. med. J.C. Gellrich
Arzt fur Orthopadie
Kriegsbergerstraße 28
D-70174 Stuttgart, Germany

Dr P. Grigoris
Senior Lecturer and Honorary Consultant
    Orthopaedic Surgeon
Department of Orthopaedic Surgery
University of Glasgow
Glasgow, UK

Professor Dr U. Gross
Universitatsklinikum Benjamin Franklin
Abteilung fur Pathologie
Hindenburgdamm 30
D-12200 Berlin, Germany

Dr W.O. Haggard
Wright Bio-Orthopaedics
5677 Airline Road
Arlington
Tennessee TN 38002, USA

Professor R. Huiskes
Professor of Musculoskeletal Biomechanics
Orthopaedic Research Laboratory
University of Nijmegan
Th. Craanenlaan 7
PO Box 9101
6500 HB Nijmegan, The Netherlands

Dr E. Ingham
Reader in Medical Immunology
Medical and Biological Engineering Group
Department of Microbiology
University of Leeds, Leeds LS2 9JT, UK

Professor T. Judet
Service Chirurgie Général II
Traumatologie et Orthopedie
Hôpital Tenon, 4 rue de la Chine
75970 Paris Cedex 20, France

Professor I.D. Learmonth
Department of Orthopaedic Surgery
Level 5
Bristol Royal Infirmary
Bristol BS2 8HW, UK

Dr A.C. Lee
School of Engineering
University of Exeter
North Park Road
Exeter EX4 4QF, UK

Mr A. McCaskie
Department of Trauma and Orthopaedic
    Surgery
The Medical School
University of Newcastle
Newcastle upon Tyne NE2 4HH, UK

Mr H. Minakawa
Research Student
Medical and Biological Engineering Group
Department of Microbiology
University of Leeds, Leeds LS2 9JT, UK

Dr R. Nizard
Hôpital Lariboisière
2 rue Ambroise Paré
75475 Paris Cedex 10, France

Dr J.E. Parr
Vice Chairman, Chief Scientific Officer and
    President
Wright Bio-Orthopaedics
5677 Airline Road
Arlington
Tennessee TN 38002, USA

Dr P. Pirou
Service Chirurgie Général II
Traumatologie et Orthopedie
Hôpital Tenon, 4 rue de la Chine
75970 Paris Cedex 20, France

Mr P. Roberts
Consultant Orthopaedic Surgeon
Royal Gwent Hospital
Cardiff Hospital
Newport, Gwent NP9 2UB, UK

Professor L. Sedel
Senior Orthopaedic Surgeon
Hôpital Lariboisière
2 rue Ambroise Paré
75475 Paris Cedex 10, France

Mr M.H. Stone
Consultant Orthopaedic Surgeon
Medical and Biological Engineering Group
Department of Orthopaedic Surgery
Leeds General Infirmary, Leeds LS1 3EX, UK

Dr J.L. Tipper
Research Fellow
Medical and Biological Engineering Group
Department of Microbiology
University of Leeds, Leeds LS2 9JT, UK

Dr H.H. Trieu
Wright Bio-Orthopaedics
5677 Airline Road
Arlington
Tennessee TN 38002, USA

Dr N. Verdonschot
Director of Implant Biomechanics
Orthopaedic Research Laboratory
University of Nijmegan
Th. Craanenlaan 7
PO Box 9101
6500 HB Nijmegan, The Netherlands

Professor Dr med. Dr. h.c. mult. S. Weller
ehem. Arztlicher Direktor der BG-Unfallklinik
    und Ordinarius fur Unfallchirurgie
Eberhard-Karls-Universitat Tubingen
Engelfriedshalde 47
D-72076 Tubingen

Professor Dr med H.-G. Willert
Orthopaedic Hospital
University of Göttingen
Robert-Koch-Straße 40
D-37075 Gottingen, Germany

Professor J. Witvoet
Hôpital Lariboisière
2 rue Ambroise Paré
75475 Paris Cedex 10, France

Professor B.M. Wroblewski
Professor of Orthopaedic Biomechanics
Centre for Hip Surgery
Wrightington Hospital
Wigan WN6 9EP, UK

Section I

Component–Cement Interface

1. Titanium Femoral Component Fixation and Experience with a Cemented Titanium Prosthesis

G. Charnley, T. Judet, P. Pirou and C. Garreau de Loubresse

Introduction

In 1791 the Reverend Gregor discovered a black magnetic sand with an unknown "elemental oxide" in Cornwall in the south-west of England. He suggested that this element should be called "Menaccanite" as it had been found near the village of Menaccan. At the same time in Germany the chemist, Klaproth found a similar mineral and referring to the mythological children of Mother Earth named it "Titanium" after the "Titans" [1, 2].

Titanium occurs mainly as the ores ilmenite ($FeTiO_3$) and rutile (TiO_2) and in these forms occupies some 0.7% of the earth's crust [3]. It was not until after the Second World War that research began into developing its potential in implant technology with the first clinical application of pure titanium being the production of screws and plates for bone fracture fixation by Leventhal in 1951 [4].

By the mid-1950s Down Brothers, in the United Kingdom, began further trials with titanium and its alloys of greater strength, which could be used in the manufacture of total hip arthroplasties as well as other orthopaedic devices [1]. They and other companies made further progress leading to uncemented fixation of orthodontic implants and cemented and uncemented total hip arthroplasty designs by the late 1970s and early 1980s [5–8].

Murray and colleagues in 1995 reviewed 62 total hip arthroplasties then available in the United Kingdom, many without long-term or even short-term clinical follow up [9]. Amongst these 27 of the femoral components were available uniquely made of titanium or as a titanium option, with 14 for cementless fixation, 5 for use with or without cement and 8 designs for insertion with acrylic bone cement.

The majority of these implants had only entered the "hip market" from the mid-1980s.

Chemical Composition, Microstructure and Biomechanical Properties

The rapid rise of titanium as one of the most common metals used for the production of hip prostheses is explained by some of its chemical and mechanical properties. It is biocompatible and was thought initially to be inert, that is to generate a low immune response. In comparison with other metals such as stainless steel or the alloys of cobalt–chrome it is more able to withstand corrosion. This ability to resist corrosion is due to a passive oxide film that forms over the surface of titanium or titanium alloys. The film develops following exposure to oxygen giving particular protection against crevice and stress corrosion [1, 3, 7, 8, 10].

Titanium has a low modulus of elasticity, which is approximately one-third to one-half that of stainless steel and cobalt–chrome. Whilst being greater than human cortical bone such reduced elasticity may lower the stress shielding of the surrounding tissue leading in turn to decreased cortical bone remodelling and resorption [10, 11]. Unfortunately titanium is sensitive to surface flaws such as notching, which may accelerate fatigue of the implants. This is one of the factors that has led to its use for femoral head components being abandoned [12].

There are alloys of titanium available along with commercially pure titanium (cP-Ti). Several grades

3

of commercially pure titanium exist with varying traces of oxygen, nitrogen, hydrogen, iron and carbon. Whilst having high corrosion resistance and proving successful in osseo-integration, the pure form is rather ductile and thus is not as strong at withstanding bending stresses when compared with its alloys or those of cobalt–chrome [1, 4, 6, 7, 10, 11].

Titanium alloy Ti-6Al-4V (ASTM F-136) is the most commonly used alloy of titanium both in Europe and the United States. Its combination with both aluminium and vanadium provides a higher yield strength with great tensile strength combined with good corrosion resistance. Ti-6Al-4V is considered a "super alloy" because of its high strength and fatigue resistance. It has two phases, an alpha phase and a beta phase, producing a so called bimodal microstructure. The alpha phase is stable at high temperatures and the beta phase at lower temperatures. In different phases the microcomposition has a granular or crystal structure [1, 7, 10, 11]. The ability to alter the relationship between these two phases by chemical and thermal manipulation provides enhanced mechanical properties. Other titanium alloys have been used in hip arthroplasty including Ti-6Al-7Nb, in which niobium replaces vanadium [7, 10, 11].

Surface Finishes

The expansion in the use of titanium coincided with varying ideas on how to improve the bonding between the cement mantle and the prosthesis or to allow a controlled subsidence of the stem within the cement mantle. Harris suggested that an improved stem fixation could be achieved by "precoating" the components with a thin layer of polymethylmethacrylate bone cement [13].

Varying femoral component designs have included many different surface finishes. Crowninshield and colleagues in 1998 classified these surface finishes for cemented femoral stems [14]. Those with the lowest surface roughness, (measured in R_a), have shiny surfaces achieved by polishing, or with slightly greater surface roughness by machining or blasting with glass beads. Such finishes may create a "compressive skin" leading to improved titanium fatigue strength. Matt and rougher surfaces are manufactured by coarser blasting with sand or grit.

For cementless fixation titanium femoral components have been modified by the surface application of plasma-sprayed alloys, sintered beads, alloy meshes and hydroxyapatite coatings on part or all of the stems. All of these surface modifications are directed at osseo-integration of the femoral

component [5, 8] and so enhance the initial stability provided by instrumentation and stem geometry.

Cementless Fixation and Osseo-integration

The father of the senior author designed one of the earliest forms of cementless hip arthroplasty. This prosthesis had large macrotexturing on the surface for initial fixation and subsequent bone ingrowth.

The term osseo-integration was coined after work by Branemark and colleagues in 1977 who demonstrated implant fixation of orthodontic titanium devices following research in Gothenburg [5, 15]. The initial encouraging fixation of these implants in the jaw led to further developments in hip surgery aiming to achieve rigid fixation of the component within the host bone, which would be maintained during functional loading [5, 8, 15].

In North America, in particular, with concern about the longevity of cemented prostheses in the younger patient, cementless prostheses evolved. In 1975 titanium stems were approved for use in the USA and there have been advocates for various femoral designs. These have included a tight diaphyseal fit with a large cylindrical prosthesis such as Engh's AML prosthesis (DuPuy, Warsaw, IN, USA) [16]. Other authors have been concerned that such devices whilst fitting and filling the femoral diaphysis may lead to proximal femoral resorption secondary to proximal stress shielding. Mallory and Head, amongst others, have preferred a proximally coated, tapered wedge design creating a mechanical interface, which as it subsides, maintains hoop stresses between itself and the bone [17]. If the coating is confined to the metaphysis it must be circumferential to avoid uncoated areas allowing access for wear debris to pass distally [18]. Good medium-term and some long-term successes have been reported by Bourne and Rorabeck, Rothman and others using proximally coated titanium alloy, ingrowth prostheses [19–22]. Equally, Zweymuller has reported encouraging results with a stem of rectangular cross-section that provides initial "three-dimensional anchorage" [23].

Biocompatibility

When titanium was initially studied it seemed to generate very little host response. Much of this early research was limited as it was purely macroscopic and relied simply on reviewing the local tissue reaction in animal models to blocks of titanium or its alloys or short-term review of simple implants such as plates and screws without wear. Bothe noted a simple fibrous membrane around implants in a rabbit model in the earliest recorded study [24].

As implant research advanced, so did the microscopic and histochemical assessment of the host response to foreign bodies including titanium prostheses. Studies in various centres have shown that particulate titanium may be present both in the periprosthetic membrane and areas of osteolysis around loose prostheses. The titanium debris may be responsible for exciting a phagocytic response via various cell mediators and titanium particles and ions may spread into the serum and urine of animal models as well as patients [25, 26].

Rae in 1975 noted that unlike cobalt and nickel, titanium metal particles generated only slight enzymatic responses in murine peritoneal macrophages [27]. By 1984 Woodman had found evidence of titanium ions in the lungs, muscle, spleen and lymph nodes of baboons [28].

In 1988 Agins studied the pseudocapsule around nine failed Ti-6Al-4V prostheses, eight of which had been cemented. There was metallic staining of the soft tissues and histiocyte and plasma cell reaction. The highest concentration of titanium was found in a cementless case where titanium wire mesh had been used for fixation [29]. Others, including Langkammer and Urban, also found that in humans titanium and titanium alloys were present in histiocytes, and at distant locations including the para-aortic lymph nodes, the liver and spleens of patients who had previously undergone hip arthroplasty [30, 31]. Hasselman and colleagues reported that titanium elicited a high mediator response in canine macrophages producing prostaglandins (PGE$_2$), in comparison with controls but this response was less than that with ultra-high-molecular-weight polyethylene [32]. Bullough's 1994 editorial entitled "Metallosis" in the *Journal of Bone and Joint Surgery* voiced concern about the potential harm of metallic debris following the failure of titanium and non-titanium arthroplasties; such concern included the risk of carcinogenesis [33].

More recent research has suggested that in the absence of wear titanium alloys may not be detrimental to the host. Goodman and co-workers reviewed the histomorphological reaction of bone to different concentrations of highly phagocytosable particles of Ti-6Al-4V and high-density polyethylene using a rabbit animal model, with long bone trauma. They found that whilst titanium provoked a histiocyte reaction it did not disturb the normal healing responses nor new bone formation [34]. Bessho et al. assessed titanium ions eluted from pure titanium miniplates in a long-term study [35]. At a minimum of 2 years post-implantation the plates showed negligible corrosion and whilst titanium was noted in organs at a distance, in particular the lungs, the levels of titanium reached a maximum at 3 months and gradually reduced over a 2-year period. Their work suggested that the ions may be eluted once the protective oxide film is lost from the surface of an implant, but eventually the excretion rate of titanium exceeds the amount released from the implant. Finally, Bianco et al. monitored titanium in the serum and urine levels of rabbits with a titanium mesh and no wear. Compared with a control group which had no titanium inserted, no difference in the titanium levels was found between each group [36].

This evolving work at a cellular and chemical basic science level suggests that titanium femoral components, whether cementless or cemented, may not be harmful in the absence of component wear. Concern, however, remains that when prostheses fail excessive particles of titanium or its alloys can be generated and may enter the local soft tissues or be spread by the reticuloendothelial system to distant organs.

Experience with a Cemented Titanium Prosthesis – the Fare Total Hip Arthroplasty

Introduction – Materials and Methods

Our experience using a cemented titanium prosthesis commenced in 1987, with the Fare total hip replacement (ICP, Chaumont, France). The prosthesis was manufactured from titanium alloy Ti-6Al-4V that also included traces of iron, oxygen, carbon, nitrogen and hydrogen. The prosthesis has a curved design with a small collar and a neck shaft angle of 135∞. It is oval in cross-section to maximize the fit and fill of the femoral medullary canal. In the review period reported it was inserted by surgeons with varying levels of experience using second-generation cementing techniques.

The use of this component was associated with early good results, with the cemented fixation providing excellent early pain relief and restoring function (Merle D'Aubigné score 12 points). However, this success was not maintained in a cohort of patients beyond a few months. Failure was noted in several cases and presented with subsidence and distal migration of the prosthesis and in other cases it was associated with the development of isolated osteolytic granulomas (Figs 1.1 and 1.2).

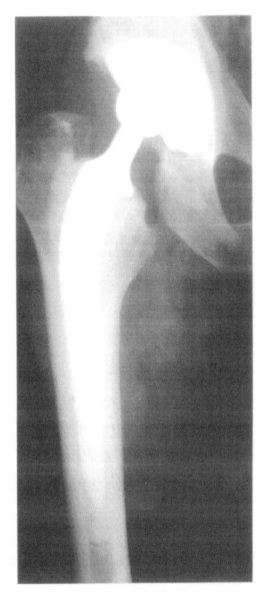

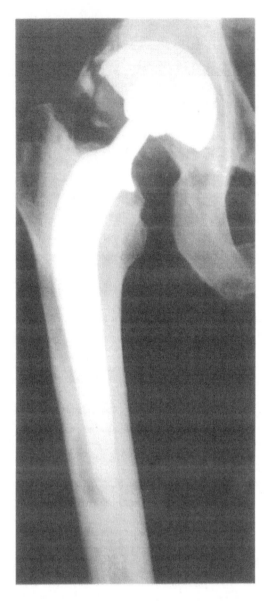

Fig. 1.1. The initial postoperative appearance of a Fare hybrid cemented hip replacement.

Fig. 1.2. Granuloma development seen radiologically on a 9-month postoperative X-ray.

These precocious failures concerned us and thus we have reviewed systematically the first 1000 Fare total hip replacements implanted. In our series we wished to assess what problems had occurred between the titanium stem and the cement.

Results

In 1997 we reviewed the first 1000 Fare total hip replacements inserted over a 6-year period between 1987 and 1993. The study excluded all patients who had had previous prosthetic surgery but included some patients who had had earlier surgery such as previous osteosynthesis for femoral neck fracture. The maximum period of review was 10 years with a median follow up of 5 years and a mean recall of 6 years.

All the patients received a questionnaire assessing their functional outcome and all were reviewed by clinical examination along with assessment of their X-rays. Out of the initial 1000 cases there were 11 patients lost to review (1.1% of the series), and a further 118 had died at the time of review from unrelated causes (12% of the series).

Table 1.1. Revision rates using the Fare total hip replacement 1987–1993

	Femoral component loosening	Osteolytic granuloma cases	Revision for infection	Other causes
1987	2	1	1	0
1988	3	3	1	0
1989	3	8	1	2
1990	2	12	1	2
1991	0	7	0	0
1992	1	1	0	0
1993	0	2	1	1

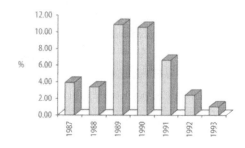

Revision rate (percentage) per year of study

Fig. 1.4. Overall revision rate (percentage) for all causes per year of study.

The overall survival curve was 90% for the total series (between 88 and 98% with a confidence interval of 5%). These results compare with early Charnley prostheses over a similar period as recorded in outcome studies such as the Swedish Hip Register [37]. However, amongst the patients available for review 53 (5.3%) had had revision surgery. After retrospective analysis four particular modes of failure were determined: pure femoral subsidence; osteolytic granuloma and loosening; acetabular component failure; and infection. The respective revision rates for all causes between 1987 and 1993 are illustrated in Table 1.1.

Figure 1.3 shows the total number of prostheses implanted year on year between 1987 and 1993 and Fig. 1.4 reveals the number of revisions for all reasons by year of implantation and is displayed as a percentage of the total number of prostheses performed in any year. The asymmetric distribution of the revision rate will be discussed later.

The following sequence of events was noted in those hips that failed. During the first 3 months no patients had any complaints and all seemed to be functioning well without pain. However, several of

these patients between the 6th and 8th postoperative month developed thigh pain and subsequent radiological investigation revealed signs of failure commonly between the 10th and 14th postoperative month. Some patients were asymptomatic, but fortuitously X-ray investigation revealed the presence of osteolytic granuloma appearing around the prosthesis. These lesions were usually solitary but often led to secondary loosening of the femoral stem.

From our radiological assessment of the failed cases, there were two types of femoral failure: these were pure femoral stem subsidence and secondary loosening due to initial osteolytic granuloma formation around the femoral stem. Histological examination of the granulomata in 12 cases of revision demonstrated titanium metallic particles with a local histiocyte response. Such granulomata were also present in cases that had not undergone revision and the total number of patients within our series, whether revised or not, who developed a granuloma has been calculated at 5.8%. The incidence of these lesions was also asymmetrical in its distribution within the period studied (Fig. 1.5). Such asymmetry matched the asymmetry of the revision surgery performed. The development of the osteolytic granulomata relative to the year of prosthetic implantation is displayed in Fig. 1.6.

When the results were subjected to survival analysis, stratified by year and reviewed in conjunction

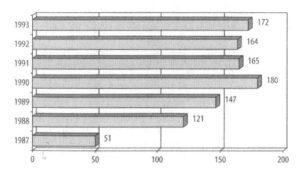

Fare total hip replacement implantation rate

1993	172
1992	164
1991	165
1990	180
1989	147
1988	121
1987	51

Fig. 1.3. Fare total hip replacement implantation rate between 1987 and 1993.

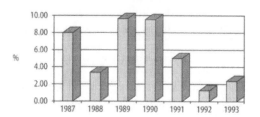

Annual rate of osteolytic granuloma presentation

Fig. 1.5. Annual rate of osteolytic granuloma presentation.

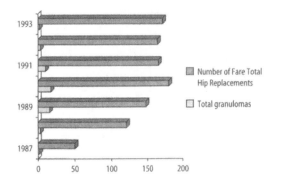

Fig. 1.6. Granuloma rate in relation to rate of Fare arthroplasty implantations.

with decreased function and the date of osteolytic lesion development we determined possible co-factors that we believed were responsible for the eventual failure of the prosthesis. During this period we had not altered our surgical technique, nor had the component geometry changed, but retrospectively we found that the cement type used and the surface finish of the component had been modified.

Between August 1983 and March 1989 the femoral component was sand blasted with glass balls and between March 1989 and April 1993 the surface finish was sandblasted with corindon beads. At the end of April 1992 the surface of the prosthesis became polished rather than sandblasted and around the same time (in February 1992) the use of Sulfix cement (Sulzer Orthopaedics, Baar, Switzerland) was discontinued. CMW cement (DePuy, Blackpool, UK) was used in its place by those surgeons inserting the implant.

When we compared the annual rate of granulomata development in relation to the surface finish of the prosthesis, (sandblasted versus smooth finish), a threefold increase in stem failure and granuloma linked to the rough surface finish was found. Statistically it was not possible to identify a different failure rate comparing the rough and smooth surfaces finishes with the different types of cements used. This is probably attributable to the fact that Sulfix cement was only used for a 2-month period before the new cement (CMW) was introduced. The period of study was too short to provide any statistical analysis of the influence of cement type independent of the change of surface finish.

Fare Hip Arthroplasty Conclusions

The initial design of the Fare total hip replacement with a rough surface finish cemented in place with Sulfix cement was associated with an incidence of osteolysis and granuloma formation of almost 10%

and an unacceptably high revision rate. The concern about osteolysis and the risk of early prosthetic failure remained, however, and from September of 1996 the Fare femoral component has been manufactured from polished stainless steel. This new stem used with modern, third-generation cementing techniques is now undergoing clinical review.

Discussion – is There a Place for a Cemented Titanium Stem?

Our early results with a rough surfaced titanium prosthesis have not been good in the long term when compared with stems of other materials or original prosthetic design such as the Charnley Low Friction Arthroplasty. Other authors using titanium or titanium alloy stems with rough surfaces and cemented fixation have had similar problems. Witt and Swann reported a high incidence of osteolysis and failure with a coarse, shot blasted Ti-6Al-4V prosthesis [38]. In accordance with our results their replacements seemed to be performing well at 6 months but between this period and 3 years clinical examination and X-rays demonstrated loosening and granuloma formation leading to component revision. Histological review of the failures found titanium in the soft tissues. These particles excited a fibroblast and giant cell reaction in the surrounding fibrous tissue. More recently the results of a "Charnley type" prosthesis inserted in Nottingham in England, were reported by Massoud and co-workers in 1997 [39]. At a mean follow up of 26 months, 26% of 76 hip replacements manufactured from a titanium alloy were clinically or radiologically loose. This high failure rate was attributed to several factors including a rough titanium surface on the stem, the scratch sensitivity of the titanium nitride head and an inadequate cement mantle. Massoud believed that the titanium alloy was particularly susceptible to abrasive wear by particles of polymethylmethacrylate once there was loosening between the prosthesis and the bone cement.

This experience has not been shared by all surgeons and some have reported good mid- and long-term results with cemented titanium stems. In an early report Sarmiento and Gruen [40] compared their 5-year results of a "Charnley" stem manufactured from titanium alloy with a similar design in steel or cobalt–chrome. They reported a lower loosening rate and lower rate of radiological resorption of the calcar with the titanium stems in comparison with other designs. This has been supported by more recent research of Cohen and Rushton who found up to 8% proximal bone resorption at a year following the use of a steel Charnley component [41].

More impressively perhaps are the early and long-term results of a cemented, smooth, titanium femoral stem combined with a modular ceramic head and a ceramic acetabular component. Witvoet and colleagues have reported excellent survival figures in patients under 50 years of age beyond 10 years [42–44].

If failure of titanium stems is reviewed, it should be noted that in the early years following its use in hip arthroplasty, many stems were monobloc or had modular titanium heads. Titanium wear debris from the head rather than the stem seems to have led to early revision. Even Agins could not determine in his paper whether the titanium stem failure was secondary to loosening and wear products from elsewhere. McKellop et al. reviewed 20 failed titanium cemented prosthesis of an early generation stem, at between 12 and 136 months, and found only low levels of titanium in the tissues where there was an absence of cement particle debris [45]. More recently Nimoniya et al. studied the induction of gene expression and protein synthesis for mediators of bone resorption on a variety of orthopaedic implant surfaces. Interleukin-6 (IL-6) was noted in response to different surfaces of titanium alloy and grit blasted surfaces produced more IL-6 than smooth surfaces. The authors postulated that IL-6 in high levels may lead to enhanced bone resorption and early implant failure [46].

Finally if we assess current practice, a 1998 review of the use of cemented stems at the American Academy of Orthopaedic Surgeons identified that 70% of the delegates preferred a smooth stem if cement were used, although no preference in material was recorded. Less than 20% favoured rough surfaces with cement and very few would now consider precoated stems [47].

Conclusion

In conclusion, it would seem reasonable to use titanium femoral stems with modern day, third-generation cementing techniques. However, the surface finish must be smooth and titanium should not be used for the bearing surface. If the component is stable with an intact cement mantle, there is less chance of titanium debris or ions being transmitted to distant sites with the previously identified concerns. This is because the titanium is shielded from the host bone and reticuloendothelial system by the surrounding cement mantle. In effect such intimate apposition between stem and cement and an intact mantle seals the potential peri-prosthetic joint space described by Schmalzried et al. [48].

Conversely, work by Chang et al. (1988) suggested that a titanium mesh with a rougher surface proved better at osseo-integration than a plasma-sprayed or smooth titanium surfaces, with implications for cementless titanium fixation [49]. Their work echoed that of Feighan et al. who found more extensive bone growth on blasted titanium stems than smooth ones [50].

However the further development of any prosthesis, whether titanium or not, and with or without cement, must be accompanied by greater surveillance during its introduction if we are to avoid the errors of the past. Initial trials should be restricted to limited centres with the results being compared with other outcomes such as those provided by national hip registers [51]. Any new prosthesis must also avoid the earlier pitfalls of changing any one of multiple variables, e.g. stem geometry; surface finish; cementing technique; head size and type and modularity, etc. in the early years following the introduction of the implant as this compromises objective review of clinical results and meaningful analysis of failures.

Acknowledgements

I am grateful for the assistance of the preparation of this chapter to Philip Cleary of Aesculap, Dr Warren MacDonald of the Department of Biomaterials/Handicap Research, Gothenburg University, Sweden, and Dr John Bradley of Orthodesign UK.

References

1. Down Brothers and Mayer and Phelps Ltd. Titanium in relation to surgery. London: Wyvern Press and Studio, 1963.
2. Gray R. The Greek myths. Harmondsworth: Penguin Books, 1995.
3. Williams DS. Systemic aspects of bio-compatibility, Volume 1. Boca Raton, FL: CRC Press Inc., 1980.
4. Leventhal GS. Titanium and metal for surgery. J Bone Joint Surg 1951;33:473–474.
5. Albrektsson T, Branemark PI, Hansson HA, Lindstrom J. Osseo-integrated titanium implants. Requirements for ensuring a long lasting direct bone anchorage in man. Acta Orthop Scand 1981;52:155–170.
6. Dobbs HS, Scales JT. Behavior of commercial pure titanium and Ti6AL4V in orthopaedic implants. ASTM-STP 1983; 796:173–186.
7. Semlitsch M. Titanium alloys for hip joint replacements. Clin Mater 1987;2:1–13.
8. Albrektsson T, Carlsson LV, Jacobsson M, MacDonald W. Gothenburg osseo integrated hip arthroplasty. Clin Orthop 1998;352:81–98.
9. Murray DW, Carr AJ, Bulstrode CJ. Which primary total hip replacement. J Bone Joint Surg 1995;77B:520–527.
10. Dee R Mango E Hurst LC. Principles of orthopaedic practice. New York: McGraw-Hill, 1989.

11. Callagham JJ, Rosenberg AG, Rubash HE. The adult hip. Philadelphia: Lippincott-Raven, 1998.
12. Galante JO, Rostocker W. Wear in total hip prostheses. Acta Orthop Scand suppl 1973;145:1–46.
13. Harris WH. Long term results of cemented femoral stems with roughened pre-coated surfaces. Clin Orthop 1998; 355:137–143.
14. Crowninshield RD, Jennings JD, Laurent J, Maloney WJ. Cemented femoral component surface finish mechanics. Clin Orthop 1998;355:90–102.
15. Johansson CB. On tissue on reactions to metal implants. MD thesis University of Gothenburg, 1991.
16. Engh CA, Hooten JP, Zettl-Schaffer KF. Porous-coated total hip replacement. Clin Orthop 1994;298:89–96.
17. Mallory TH, Head CW, Lombardi AV. Tapered design for cementless total hip arthroplasty femoral component. Clin Orthop 1997;344:172–178.
18. Urban RM, Jacobs JJ, Sumner DR et al. The bone–implant interface of femoral stems with non-circumferential porous coating. J Bone Joint Surg 1996;78A:1068–1081.
19. Bourne RB, Rorabeck CH, Burkhart BC, Kirk PG. Ingrowth surfaces. Plasma spray coating to titanium alloy hip replacements. Clin Orthop 1994;298:37–46.
20. Bourne RB, Rorabeck CH. A critical look at cementless stems. Clin Orthop 1998;355:212–223.
21. Rothman R. Proximal coated titanium femoral prosthesis. J Bone Joint Surg 1996;78A:319–324.
22. Mont MA, Hungerford DS. Proximally coated in growth prostheses: a review. Clin Orthop 1997;344:139–149.
23. Zweymuller KA, Lintner FK, Semlitsch MF. Biological fixation of a press-fit titanium hip joint endoprosthesis. Clin Orthop 1998;235:195–206.
24. Bothe RT, Beaton LE, Davenport HA. Reaction of bone to multiple metallic implants. Surg. Gynecol Obstet 1940;71:598–602.
25. Ferguson AB, Akhoshi Y, Laing PG, Hodge ES. Characteristics of trace ions released from embedded metal implants in the rabbit. J Bone Joint Surg 1962;44A:323–336.
26. Jacobs JJ, Skipor AK, Black J, Urban RM, Galante JO. Release and excretion of metal in patients who have a total hip-replacement component made of titanium-base alloy. J Bone Joint Surg 1991;73A:1475–1486.
27. Rae T. A study of the effects of particular metals of orthopaedic interest on murine macrophages in vitro. J Bone Joint Surg 1975;57B:444–450.
28. Woodman JL, Jacobs JJ, Galante JO, Urban RM. Metal ion released from titanium–based prosthetic segmental replacements of long bones in baboons, a long term study. J Orthop Res 1984;421:430–435.
29. Agins HJ, Alcock NW, Bansal M et al. Metallic wear in failed titanium–alloy total hip replacements, a histological and quantitative analysis. J Bone Joint Surg 1988;70A:347–356.
30. Langkamer VG, Case CP, Heap P et al. Systemic distribution of wear debris after hip replacement. J Bone Joint Surg 1992;74B:831–839.
31. Urban RM, Jacobs JJ, Tomlinson MJ et al. Particles of metal alloys and their corrosion products in the liver spleen and para-aortic lymph nodes of patients with total hip replacement prostheses. Trans Orthop Res Soc 1995; Orlando, Florida.
32. Hasselman CT, Kovach CJ, Keys B, Rubash HE, Shanbhag AS. Macrophage response to synergistic challenge with prosthetic wear debris. Trans Orthop Res Soc 1997; San Francisco, California.
33. Bullough PG. Metallosis. J Bone Joint Surg 1994;76B: 687–688.
34. Goodman SP, Davidson JA, Song Y, Marshall N, Fornasier VL. Histomorphological reaction of bone to different concentrations of high phagocytosable particles of high density polyethylene and Ti 6AL-4V alloy in vitro. Trans Orthop Res Soc 1997; San Francisco, California.
35. Bessho K, Fujimura K, Iizuka T. Experimental long-term study of titanium irons eluted from pure titanium mini plates. J Biomed Mater Res 1995;29:901–904.
36. Bianco PD, Ducheyne P, Cuckler JM. Titanium serum and urine levels in rabbits with a titanium implant in the absence of wear. J Biomater 1996;17:1937–1942.
37. Herberts P, Malchau H. Prognosis of total hip replacement. Scientific Exhibition presented at the 63rd Annual Meeting of the American Academy of Orthopedic Surgeons, Atlanta, USA,1996.
38. Witt JD, Swann M. Metalwear and tissue response in failed titanium alloy total hip replacements. J Bone Joint Surg 1991;73B:559–563.
39. Massoud SN, Hunter JB, Houldsworth BJ, Wallace WA, Juliusson R. Early femoral loosening in one design of cemented hip replacement. J Bone Joint Surg 1997;99B: 603–608.
40. Sarmiento A, Gruen TA. Radiographic analysis of a low modulus titanium alloy femoral total hip component. J Bone Joint Surg 1985;67A:48–53.
41. Cohen B, Rushton N. Bone remodeling in the proximal femur after Charnley total hip arthroplasty. J Bone Joint Surg 1995;77B:815–819.
42. Sedel L, Kerboull L, Christel P, Meunier A, Witvoet J. Alumina on alumina hip replacement. Results and survivorship in young patients. J Bone Joint Surg 1990;72B:653–658.
43. Nizard RS, Sedel L, Christel P, Meunier A, Soudry M, Witvoet J. Ten year survivorship of cemented ceramic–ceramic total hip prosthesis. Clin Orthop 1992;282:53–63.
44. Sedel L, Nizard RS, Kerboull L, Witvoet J. Alumina–alumina hip replacement in patients younger than 50 years old. Clin Orthop 1994;298:175–183.
45. McKellop, HA, Sarmiento A, Schwinn CP, Edramzadeh E. In vivo wear of titanium-alloy hip prostheses. J Bone Joint Surg 1990;72A 512–517.
46. Ninomiya JT, Struve JA, Abel SM, Shetty RH, Lin SD. Orthopaedic Implant surfaces induce gene expression and protein synthesis for mediators of bone resorption. Trans Orthop Res Soc 1997; San Francisco, California
47. Cemented Stem Review. 1998 meeting of the American Academy of Orthopaedic Surgeons New Orleans, USA, 1998.
48. Schmalried TP, Jasty M, Harris WH. Periprosthetic bone loss in total hip arthroplasty. J Bone Joint Surg 1992; 74A:849–863.
49. Change Y-S, Gu H-O, Kobayashim et al. Influence of various structure treatments on histological fixation of titanium implants. J Bone Joint Surg 1988; 70A:347–356.
50. Feighan JE, Goldberg M, Dwight D, Parr J, Stevenson S. The influence of surface-blasting on the incorporation of titanium-alloy implants in a rabbit intramedullary model. J Bone Joint Surg 1995;77A:1380–1395.
51. Grigoris P, Hamblen D. The control of new prosthetic implants. J Bone Joint Surg 1998;80B:941–943.

2. The Time-dependent Properties of Polymethylmethacrylate Bone Cement: the Interaction of Shape of Femoral Stems, Surface Finish and Bone Cement

A.J.C. Lee

Introduction

Polymethylmethacrylate (PMMA) bone cement has been used to fix implants into bones in humans for more than 30 years. It is, perhaps, the least well understood of the implant components – it has been blamed for early failure, it has been called the "weak link" in the replacement joint system, etc. In order for bone cement to be used successfully in long-term fixation of a total replacement hip joint, the femoral and acetabular components must be designed to take account of the properties of the bone cement and the surgeon must use a surgical (cementing) technique that ensures good quality cement and good quality interfaces between cement and stem or cup, and cement and bone. This chapter will consider the properties of PMMA bone cement and discuss how these properties interact with the shape and surface finish of a total hip femoral stem to alter the way in which load is transmitted across the cement–stem and cement–bone interfaces.

Nature and Structure of PMMA Bone Cement

In order to understand the physical behaviour of polymethylmethacrylate bone cement in a total joint replacement, it is necessary to understand the basic nature and structure of the material [1]. PMMA bone cement is a polymer made up of long-chain molecules containing many thousands of "elements" (monomers). The long-chain molecules are wound around each other in an unstructured manner (it has an amorphous structure) and consist of strongly bonded covalent chains with side groups that are linked by relatively weaker secondary bonds. Bone cement is a thermoplastic polymer, that is, its behaviour and properties vary as the temperature of the polymer varies. The temperature most often quoted in text books is the glass transition temperature. Above this temperature (about 95 °C for bone cement) the polymer has a much lower apparent modulus, with the long chain molecules more free to slide over each other giving the polymer leathery properties. There are other transitions (secondary transitions) which are important, and for bone cement one of these occurs at about 25 °C – above room temperature but below body temperature. The secondary transition is a result of the relaxation of the weaker secondary bonds between the side groups, allowing the side groups to flick over each other. The effect of this transition is that bone cement is much more flexible in the body than it is at room temperature (Fig. 2.1a, b). The consequence of the temperature dependency of PMMA bone cement is that any tests which are designed to show how bone cement performs in an implant system must be carried out at body temperature (37 °C) or slightly higher.

Short-term Mechanical Properties of PMMA Bone Cement

Short-term mechanical properties of bone cement are well known and are easily found by taking samples of cement into a testing laboratory and testing in a conventional materials test machine. Typical values for PMMA bone cement [2–5] show it has a relatively high compressive strength (about

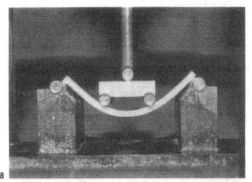

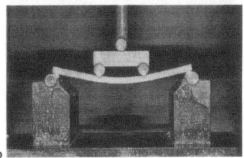

Fig. 2.1. **a** Beam of bone cement under a standard load for 24 hours at 37 °C. **b** Beam of bone cement under the same load as **a** for 24 hours at 18 °C.

90 MPa), a medium shear strength (about 50 MPa) and a relatively low tensile strength (about 25 MPa). The modulus of elasticity (Young's modulus) is normally obtained from a tension test and is the ratio of stress to strain (most often calculated as the ratio of load to extension) in the elastic region. The modulus of elasticity of bone cement is about 2400 MPa. This is a low value compared with the modulus of the other materials which surround the cement in a replacement joint – cortical bone has a modulus about 10× and the stainless steel or cobalt–chrome alloy used for the femoral component a modulus about 100× that of bone cement. Consequently, the conventional short-term mechanical properties of bone cement tell us that it is a material which should be used in compression and protected from tension, and that it is a soft interlayer between two relatively hard layers.

Long-Term Mechanical Properties of PMMA Bone Cement

Since bone cement is a polymer which is to be used in patients for very long times (more than 20 years), the long-term properties of the material are

extremely important. The long-term properties which will be considered here are creep, stress relaxation and fatigue.

Creep is defined as time-dependent deformation under constant load. If a specimen of bone cement is loaded in tension, then it will extend at the time of loading by an amount which depends on the magnitude of the load. If the load is left in place, as time passes, the extension of the bone cement specimen will increase – the extension depends on the size of the load and the length of time it is applied. All bone cements exhibit this time dependent ability to deform; Fig. 2.2 shows creep test results for a number of commercially available bone cements. The figure plots the central deflection of a beam specimen of bone cement under four-point bending (the experimental set up is the same as that shown in Fig. 2.1). It can be seen that the polymethylmethacrylate bone cements all creep to give between 1.5 mm and 3 mm central deflection in 48 hours, however Boneloc® cement, a polybutylmethacrylate-based bone cement, creeps by about 8 mm in 10 hours. The mechanical properties of polybutylmethacrylate based bone cements are clearly not the same as those of polymethylmethacrylate based bone cements. They are different materials and care needs to be taken by surgeons when choosing a "bone cement". Although both materials may be labelled as bone cement, a surgeon must be sure that the nature of the material is appreciated; PBMA bone cement is as different from PMMA bone cement as cobalt-chrome alloy is different from titanium alloy. Simply calling both materials "bone cement" is similar to calling the cobalt-chrome or titanium alloys "metal" and being content to use a "metal" femoral stem. With polymethylmethacrylate bone cement, creep occurs most easily under tensile or shear loading, and faster when the cement is young (i.e. in the first 3 months or so). Creep is also affected by the environment (e.g. a saline or fatty environment acts as a plasticiser to cement) and occurs faster in areas of high stress [6].

Stress relaxation, the second long-term material property, is defined as change in stress level with time at constant strain. If a specimen of bone cement is put into a testing machine and put under tension, it will extend. If, before fracture takes place, the jaws of the machine are locked off and the specimen is held at constant deformation, the force to maintain the specimen in that deformed condition can be monitored with respect to time. As time passes, it will be found that the force needed to maintain the deformation reduces; dividing the force by the cross sectional area of the specimen gives stress in the specimen, so stress reduces with time at constant deformation – stress relaxation. Stress relaxation

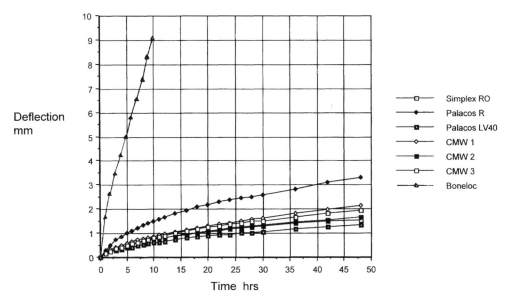

Fig. 2.2. Creep of various bone cements. Specimens 7 days old at start of tests, four-point bending, central deflection measured against time.

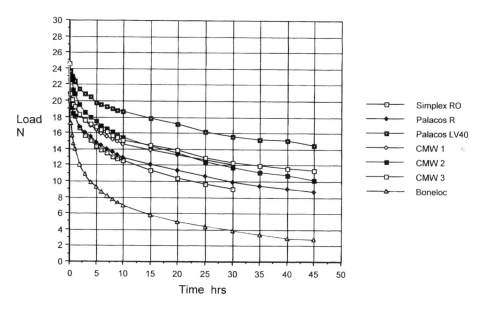

Fig. 2.3. Stress relaxation of various bone cements. Specimens 7 days old at start of tests, four-point bending, constant central deflection, load to maintain deflection measured against time.

occurs by the same mechanism in the material as that which causes creep. In both creep and stress relaxation, it is the movement between side groups, over and around each other in the long chain molecular structure of the material, which causes the material to stretch under constant load (creep) or reduce stress level under constant deformation (stress relaxation). All bone cements show the property of stress relaxation; Fig. 2.3 shows stress relaxation of a number of commercially available bone

cements tested in four-point bending with constant central deflection. It can be seen that Boneloc® bone cement exhibits faster stress relaxation than conventional PMMA bone cements, emphasising the difference between the two types of material. Like creep, stress relaxation is most significant in the face of tensile loading – tension stress reduces quickly when cement is stretched and held at constant deformation – and is affected by all the same variables that affect creep.

The final long-term property to be considered here is fatigue, defined as the cumulative effect of repeated applications of loading cycles below the level needed to cause failure with a single application of the load cycle. An unconstrained specimen of bone cement will always fail by fatigue if sufficient loading cycles are imposed in a fatigue test. However, at the stress levels found in total joints it is likely to be necessary to apply many millions of load cycles before failure takes place. Fatigue failure is usually initiated at a site of tensile stress on a surface – if the stress condition of bone cement within the implant system is maintained as primarily compressive (also advantageous from the material strength characteristics) then fatigue failure will be less likely to occur. If, in addition, the bone cement has the opportunity to stress relax (thereby reducing tensile stress levels) it will have a built in "self preservation" mechanism. Suitable design of the femoral stem of an implant can ensure that these favourable conditions exist and fatigue failure of bone cement should not be a problem.

The Significance of the Time-dependent Properties of Bone Cement

What is the significance of creep, stress relaxation and fatigue of bone cement in the transmission of load through a femoral stem?

There are three distinct types of femoral stem in common use, distinguished by their design philosophy for fixation of the stem and transmission of load. The types are:

(a) Stem fixed to the bone without bone cement.
(b) Stem fixed to bone cement which is fixed to bone.
(c) Stem acting as a taper within bone cement, cement fixed to bone.

Stem type (a) (Fig. 2.4) – the cementless stem – is fixed directly to the bone. The stem will usually have some form of surface treatment, which may take the form of sintered beads, a coating of hydroxyapatite or some other surface finish. The surface treatment may extend over the whole or part of the surface and acts to encourage ingrowth (or ongrowth) of bone to the stem surface. The stem and bone are designed to act as a composite beam, that is both will deform as a single structure with no relative movement at the interface between stem and bone. The stem has to be relatively large in section as it has to fill the femoral medullary canal. It is therefore very stiff in bending and torsion compared

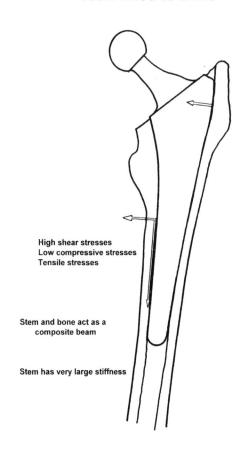

Stem fixed to bone

High shear stresses
Low compressive stresses
Tensile stresses

Stem and bone act as a
composite beam

Stem has very large stiffness

Fig. 2.4.   Stem type (a): cementless fixation of stem to bone.

with the femur. Large shear stresses are developed at the implant bone interface to carry the substantially vertical loads imposed on the implant. Relatively small radial compressive stresses are developed at the interface because they have to be generated solely as a result of the resolved component of load caused by the generally tapered shape of the stem. Since the surfaces of the stem and the bone are interlocked, there is the possibility of tensile stresses in the system due to bending, particularly at the proximal lateral interface.

Stem type (b) (Fig. 2.5) is the traditional cemented stem. Stems of this type commonly have some form of collar between neck and stem and frequently have a satin matt surface finish with a surface texture R_a value of about 1 μm. The stem is designed to be fixed to the inside surface of the bone cement, which is, in turn, fixed to the bone, so that stem, cement and bone deform as a composite beam. There is supposed to be no relative movement at the interfaces between cement and stem and between cement and bone (indeed a number of stems have been supplied precoated with PMMA to attempt to lock the interface

Stem fixed to cement

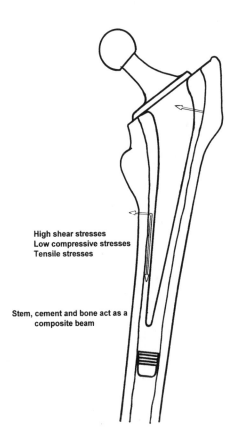

High shear stresses
Low compressive stresses
Tensile stresses

Stem, cement and bone act as a
composite beam

Fig. 2.5. Stem type (b): conventional cemented stem with a collar.

(micromovement) at the cement-stem interface is not uncommon in clinical use of this type of implant. The effect of the micromovement is to cause fretting at the interface, resulting in removal of large numbers of microparticles of metal from the surface of the stem and large quantities of particles of cement from the inside surface of the cement mantle. A satin, matt-surfaced stem removed for aseptic loosening will normally show areas of polishing when observed carefully [7–9]; the polishing confirms removal of metal from the implant surface. The generation of debris produced by fretting is difficult to control in the long term, and both metal and cement debris at the bone–cement interface can produce aseptic loosening of the stem. While the interfaces of the type b stem remain intact, the implant system will function perfectly. When the interfaces fail, by micro-movement or otherwise, significant amounts of debris are produced and the whole implant system is in danger of failure.

Stem type (c) (Fig. 2.6) is also cemented into the femoral medullary cavity, but is shaped so that it is tapered and collarless and has a highly polished

Stem moves within cement

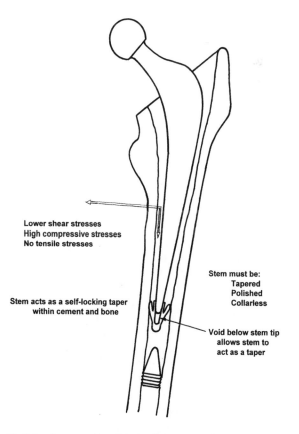

Lower shear stresses
High compressive stresses
No tensile stresses

Stem acts as a self-locking taper
within cement and bone

Stem must be:
Tapered
Polished
Collarless

Void below stem tip
allows stem to
act as a taper

Fig. 2.6. Stem type (c): polished, collarless, tapered, cemented stem.

between stem and cement permanently). In a similar way to the cementless system, high shear stresses, low compressive stresses and some tensile stresses are created at the interfaces between stem and cement and cement and bone. There are a number of potential problems with this type of fixation philosophy. The interface between cement and bone is of primary importance for the long-term survival of the implant system – if this interface fails then the whole system is likely to fail. The aim of the surgeon when inserting an implant is to make the cement-bone interface as strong as possible. To this end, lavage, cement pressurisation and a number of other cementing technique steps are followed. Unfortunately, the strength of the cement-bone interface is always limited – to the strength of the bone in the best possible case. It is not difficult to make the strength of the cement-stem interface stronger than this, using textured stems, precoated stems, etc. In these circumstances, under conditions of overload for example, there is considerable potential for the weaker cement–bone interface to fail, which would be fatal for the implant system. Relative movement surface finish with an R_a of about 0.01 μm. The combination of these design features results in the stem transmitting load to the femur differently from type (b) stems and makes specific use of the long-term material properties of creep and stress relaxation of bone cement. The coefficient of friction between a polished surface and the surrounding cement is much lower than that between a satin matt surface and cement. The result of this is that the maximum shear stress that can be developed at the stem–cement interface is much lower than that which can be developed at a high friction (matt) interface. Consequently, there will be movement at the stem–cement interface when load is put on the stem, allowing the tapered stem to subside (engage) in the cement mantle, producing radial compressive stresses and tensile hoop stresses in the mantle. The production of debris which could result from the movement of stem relative to the cement is also much lower – a smooth interface does not abrade the surface as much as a rough interface. It should be noted that, in the comparative absence of the ability to transmit shear at the stem–cement interface, the only way for the polished, collarless, tapered stem to transmit vertical load is for the stem to act as a genuine taper and engage with the cement by subsiding within it. In order to encourage the engagement of the taper without producing end bearing and punch out fractures in the cement at the stem tip, a void has to be created below the stem tip. This void can be produced by a PMMA centraliser mounted on the stem before it is inserted into the cement. The mechanism of load transmission of stems of type (c) is complicated and will be described in the following paragraph.

The stem is inserted into cement in the femur and is loaded by activity of the patient, the loads through the hip joint being transmitted to the stem, from the stem to the cement and from the cement to the bone and musculature around the joint. A "normal" patient applies about 1 million load cycles each year, therefore at least 20 million load cycles can be expected to be applied during the lifetime of a total hip replacement (THR), well into the region where fatigue failure might be expected to be important. In the case of bone cement in a patient, the cycles of load are not applied continuously but are applied, in general terms, during the time the patient is awake (about 16 hours per day) and are reduced to nearly nothing while the patient is asleep (about 8 hours per day). The cycle of generally loaded periods followed by generally unloaded periods repeats daily. With a polished, collarless, tapered femoral stem, the loads cause the stem to move within the cement – to engage the taper – the movement being accommodated by elastic deformation and creep

deformation of the cement, its surrounding bone and musculature. Each time load is applied, submicroscopic movement takes place and it is only after 3 or 4 weeks of loading that movement of the stem can be detected by X-ray or RSA (Ornstein et al. [10] measured 0.7 mm subsidence by Roentgen stereophotogrammetry (RSA) at 4 weeks postoperatively). At the end of a day's activity, some movement of the stem into the cement will have accumulated, putting strain energy into the cement and surrounding structures sufficient to support the loads which were applied. When the patient sleeps, the loading is taken off the stem which remains where it is in the cement (it has a self-locking taper). Therefore the deformation in the cement caused by loading through the stem is not recovered and the residual strain energy stored in the cement and surrounding structures is more than is needed to support the reduced load. Consequently, the stresses left in the cement, caused by the movement of the taper into the cement, are now able to be lowered by stress relaxation. It is the tensile stresses which reduce significantly, to lower the strain energy in the cement to the level needed to support the reduced loads and, incidentally, protecting the cement against fatigue failure which is normally initiated by high tensile stress. The compressive stresses and the shear stresses in the cement are not affected as much as the tensile stresses and may be assumed to remain approximately at the "loaded" level. When the patient wakes up next day, activity recommences and the stem is loaded again. The strain energy in the cement and surrounding structures needs to be increased from the "rest" level to the "activity" level. This is accomplished by more movement of the stem into the cement, expanding and compressing it to set up approximately the previous level of tensile stress and higher levels of compressive stress in the cement. The cycle of loading, micromovement of the stem and creation of stresses in the cement, followed by unloading, during which stress reduction without movement of the stem occurs, is repeated daily, accumulating movement of the stem in the cement without increasing harmful tensile stresses in the cement (Fig. 2.7). The amount of movement of the stem in the cement gets smaller as time passes since engagement of the stem causes the cement to expand outwards where it is constrained more and more by the cortical bone of the femoral shaft. Additionally, the creep rate of the cement gets smaller with time and stress levels in the cement become generally lower and more uniform giving yet lower rates of creep.

```
┌─────────────────────────────────────────────────────────┐
│        Patient awake and active, Loads applied           │
│                          ↓                               │
│   Stem moves within cement to engage the taper, giving    │
│  compressive stresses, hoop tensile stresses, shear stresses. │
│   Strain energy level at that needed to support applied loads │
│                          ↓                               │
│        Patient asleep and inactive, Loads reduced         │
│                          ↓                               │
│   Stem remains in position, strain energy still at high level, │
│                  leaving residual stresses               │
│                          ↓                               │
│  Hoop tension stresses lowered by stress relaxation, reducing │
│    strain energy to lower level to support reduced load   │
│                          ↓                               │
│        Patient awake and active, Loads applied           │
│                     Cycle repeats                         │
└─────────────────────────────────────────────────────────┘
```

Fig. 2.7. Pattern of loading, strain energy and stresses during a 24-hour period.

Clinical and Laboratory Evidence of the Effect of Stem Geometry and Surface Finish

There is some clinical and laboratory evidence that surface finish and stem geometry affect stem performance in the way described above. In a series of tests in the laboratory with polished, circular cross section metal tapers in cylinders of bone cement, the movement of the tapers into the cement when under vertical load at 37 °C was measured [11]. The results of these experiments are summarised in Fig. 2.8. It can be seen that a taper under a continuous vertical load of 196.2 N (20 kg) subsided by about 1.75 mm in 80 hours inside an unconstrained mantle of cement. When a load pattern of six hours under a load of 196.2 N (20 kg) followed by 18 hours at a reduced load of 9.8 N (1 kg) was applied, the taper subsided a total of 3.5 mm when the cement was not constrained and by 2.75 mm when the cement was constrained by a thin metal shell. The pattern of subsidence was changed by the pattern of loading; it is postulated that the difference is due to stress relaxation in the cement during periods of unloading as described in Fig. 2.7.

The clinical behaviour of cemented tapered polished collarless stems of type (c) and cemented collared matt stems of type (b) has been investigated by RSA. The first investigation [10] studied the pattern of movement of five Exeter (type (c)) stems, with tantalum markers set into the cement and the bone of the femur. In two of these cases the contrast between the markers and the cement allowed RSA to measure the movement of the stem, cement and bone with respect to each other. In both of these cases the stem moved with respect to the cement, but the cement did not move with respect to the bone. In the second investigation [12], 13 Exeter (type (c)) stems and twelve Charnley (type (b)) stems were observed in patients over 2 years. The implants had completely different patterns of distal migration. The Exeter stems moved with respect to the cement (rapidly during the first year) but the cement did not move with respect to the bone of the femur. The Charnley stems migrated more slowly than the Exeter, with movement at the cement–stem interface and the cement–bone interface. The conclusion was reached that different designs of implants migrate at different interfaces.

The difference between the subsidence pattern due to stem surface finish alone is illustrated by clinical experience with a polished and a matt version of the Exeter stem. The early clinical experience at the Princess Elizabeth Orthopaedic Hospital, Exeter (from 1970 to 1975) was with a tapered collarless, polished stem. The period from 1976 to 1985 saw the use of a stem of the same geometry, but with a matt surface finish. The difference between the clinical results of the two implants is substantial: the aseptic loosening rate of 180 matt surfaced Exeter stems inserted at the Princess Elizabeth Orthopaedic Hospital in 1980 was almost four times the loosening rate of the original polished stems at 20 years [13–15]. The difference between the two types of stem is confirmed by the results of the Swedish Hip Registry [16, 17]. A major contributor to the difference must be the strength of the interface between cement and stem in the two stem types, matt stems of type (b) have a much stronger interface than polished stems of type (a). Thus, matt stems can transmit more shear stress across the interface, increasing the shear stress applied to the weaker cement–bone interface. Secondly, the matt stems do not move with respect to the cement as the polished stems do, therefore residual strains (and residual stresses) are not left in the cement upon unloading, consequently stress relaxation does not occur and a different pattern of stresses is built up over long periods. Finally, if movement does occur between cement and stem with matt surfaced stems, much more debris is generated at the interface than when movement occurs between polished stems and cement [18].

The differing mode of load transmission between the two types of cemented stems is further illustrated by the recent experience in Norway with Exeter

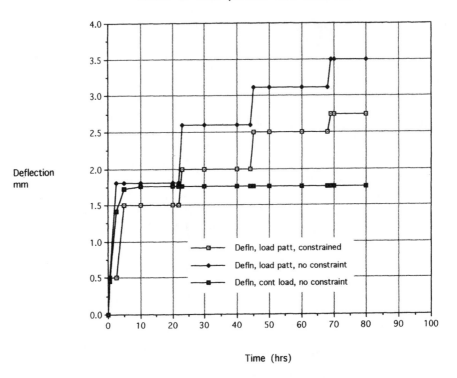

Fig. 2.8.   The effect of loading pattern and constraint on the movement of a polished taper in bone cement at 37 °C.

and Charnley stems inserted with Boneloc® (PBMA) bone cement [19]. The clinical performance of both types of stem with this cement was much less satisfactory than with PMMA bone cement, with a higher aseptic loosening rate after very short implantation times. However, the Exeter stem was affected significantly less than the Charnley; the Exeter survival rate was 97.0% at 4.5 years compared with the Charnley survival rate of 74.1% at 4.5 years (the Charnley stem has a survival rate of 98.2% and the Exeter stem a survival rate of 99.6% at 4.5 years with PMMA cement). The significant difference in survival rate between stems of the two types must result from a difference in the way each stem type loads the bone cement. The polished, collarless, tapered Exeter stem leaves residual strain in the cement when the stem is unloaded, the residual strain is caused by movement of the self-locking taper stem into the cement mantle; such stems remain in the subsided position after removal of load. The geometry of the Charnley stem, together with its surface finish, means that it does not leave significant residual strain in the cement during periods of unloading. Consequently, the opportunity for the Boneloc® cement to stress relax and reduce tensile stresses when used with the Charnley is

negligible. Since the tensile strength of Boneloc® has been reported as about half that of Palacos® bone cement [20] and the cement has been reported as fragmented when removed at revision [21], the difference in the ability of the two stems to reduce tensile stress in the cement appears to be clinically significant.

The final consequence of the difference in behaviour of polished and matt cemented stems relates to the prediction of performance using laboratory tests. In order to accelerate testing, it has become normal to test with load cycles applied at about 4 Hz (normal patient activity applies load at about 1 Hz) and with the load cycles applied continuously, with rest periods completely omitted. Thus, a typical accelerated study [22] applied 10 million load cycles (about 8 to 10 years clinical use) in 60 days of continuous loading. The absence of rest periods, during which the effects of stress relaxation can take place, means that accelerated tests such as the one referenced cannot predict clinical performance. It may not be necessary to perform tests in real time, and some acceleration of testing can be used, but the test protocol must allow periods of unloading for stress relaxation when testing polished, collarless, tapered, cemented stems.

Summary

Load transmission through the stem of a cemented THR joint depends on stem shape, stem surface finish and the properties of the cement. With a conventional, collared, matt-surfaced stem, the implant system will function well provided any movement (which may be microscopic) occurring at an interface does not produce excessive debris. Movement associated with the generation of excessive debris is a precursor of failure. With a tapered, polished, collarless stem, the stem is allowed to subside within the cement, the movement being accommodated by cycles of creep and stress relaxation in the cement. The end result of subsidence, creep and stress relaxation is to increase the compressive stress in the cement and on the cement-bone interface which should lead to long term stability of the total joint.

References

1. Ashby MF, Jones DRH. Section C: Polymers and composites. In: Engineering materials 2. Oxford: Pergamon Press, 1988; 201–240.

2. Lee AJC, Ling RSM, Vangala SS. Some clinically relevant variables affecting the mechanical behaviour of bone cement. Arch Orthop Traumat Surg 1978;92:1–18.

3. Saha S, Pal S. Mechanical properties of bone cement: a review. J Biomed Mater Res 1984;18:435–462.

4. Eyerer P, Jin R. Influence of mixing technique on some properties of PMMA bone cement. J Biomed Mater Res 1986; 20:1057–1094.

5. Lindén U. Mechanical properties of bone cement. Clin Orthop Rel Res 1991;272:274–278.

6. Lee AJC, Perkins RD, Ling RSM. Time dependent properties of polymethylmethacrylate bone cement. In: Older J (ed) Implant bone interface. Berlin: Springer-Verlag, 1990; 85–90.

7. Hale DG, Lee AJC, Ling RSM, Hooper RM. Debris production by the femoral component in cemented total hip replacement. J Bone Joint Surg 1991;73B (suppl.1):18.

8. Lee AJC, Hooper RM, Ling RSM, Brooks R, Gie GA, Hale R. Fretting as a source of particulate debris in total joint arthroplasty. In: Turner-Smith AR (ed) Micromovement in orthopaedics. Oxford: Clarendon Press, 1993; 82–98.

9. Anthony PP, Gie GA, Howie CR, Ling RSM. Localised endosteal bone lysis in relation to the femoral components of cemented total hip arthroplasties. J Bone Joint Surg 1990;72B:971–979.

10. Ornstein E, Franzén H, Johnsson R, Löfqvist T, Stefánsdottir A, Sundberg M. Does the tapered Exeter stem migrate at the stem-cement interface or/and at the cement-bone interface. Acta Orthop Scand 1997;(Suppl 274):68.

11. Hughes N, Gie GA, Lee AJC, Ling RSM. The time-dependent properties of bone cement and femoral component function. J Bone Joint Surg 1997;79B (suppl.III):367.

12. Alfaro-Adrian J, Crawford RW, Murray DW. Cement mantle migration after THR. A comparison of Charnley and Exeter with RSA. Scientific Presentation, European Orthopaedic Research Society, Amsterdam, 1988.

13. Timperley AJ, Gie GA, Lee AJC, Ling RSM. The femoral component as a taper in cemented total hip arthroplasty. J Bone Joint Surg 1993;75B (suppl.1):33.

14. Gie GA, Crawford RW, Ling RSM. An 8 to 10 year clinical review comparing matt and polished Exeter stems. J Bone Joint Surg 1998;80B (suppl.1):54.

15. Ling RSM. The history and development of the Exeter hip. London: Howmedica Inc, 1997.

16. Malchau H, Herberts P. Prognosis of total hip replacement. Scientific Exhibition, 63rd Annual Meeting, AAOS, Atlanta, USA, 1996.

17. Malchau H, Herberts P. Prognosis of total hip replacement. Revision and re-revision rate in THR: a revision risk study of 148 359 primary operations. A report from the Swedish National Hip Arthroplasty Register. Scientific Exhibition, 65th AAOS meeting, New Orleans, USA, 1998.

18. Verdonschot N. Biomechanical failure scenarios for cemented total hip replacement. PhD Thesis, Catholic University of Nijmegen, The Netherlands, 1995.

19. Furnes O, Lie SA, Havelin LI, Vollset SE, Engesaeter LB. Exeter and Charnley arthroplasties with Boneloc or high viscosity cement. Acta Orthop Scand 1997;68(6):515–520.

20. Thanner J, Freij-Larsson C, Kärrholm J, Malchau H, Wesslén B. Evaluation of Boneloc®. Acta Orthop Scand 1995; 66(3):207–214.

21. Riegels-Neilson P, Sørensen L, Andersen HM, Lindequist S. Boneloc® cemented total hip prostheses. Acta Orthop Scand 1995;66(3):215–217.

22. Davies J, Anderson MJ, Harris WH. The cement-metal interface of the Exeter stem during fatigue loading of a simulated THAA in-situ. Trans Orthop Res Soc 1996;21:525.

3. Femoral Stem Design and Cement Mantle Stress

N. Verdonschot and R. Huiskes

Introduction

This chapter will describe how the design of femoral components of cemented total hip replacements (THR) affects the stresses generated in the cement mantle. Intuitively, one would expect that cement stresses, and therefore failure, are affected by prosthetic design. However, the failure process of a cemented THR is complex, governed by component as well as patient- and surgeon-dependent variables. The question is whether there is any evidence that prosthetic design does affect the longevity of cemented THR reconstructions. An answer to this question can be found in the Scandinavian Hip Registers [1–3] which have produced a large amount of data about risk-factors that determine survival of THR reconstructions. The Registers show that significantly different survival rates are produced by different hip systems. Hence, it is very likely that prosthetic design does affect clinical outcome. The Registers also provide data about relatively small changes in the design of the hip systems and their effects on prosthetic survival. The Swedish Register [2] provides an example of how a prosthetic collar may affect prosthetic survival. With a prosthetic collar, the results of the Scan Hip prosthesis were considerably better than without it. This should not be considered as a general rule, but one that does apparently apply to the Scan Hip system. Another example of a relatively small change which affected clinical outcome is the alternative surface finish applied to the Exeter hip system a decade ago. By changing the surface finish of the femoral component from matt to polished the survival rates improved from about 88% after 9 years to about 96% after the same time period [2]. Hence, it can be concluded that different prosthetic designs produce different survival rates and that relatively small changes to a design may have a significant effect on the durability of THR reconstructions.

In this chapter we describe a few issues which need to be considered when designing a cemented femoral component. Some general principles are discussed, such as the load-transfer mechanism of prosthetic components and how it is affected by stem–cement bonding characteristics. How stem–cement bonding strength can be improved and cement mantle stresses can be reduced once stem–cement debonding has occurred is also discussed. In addition, the application of computer optimisation techniques is discussed, which can be used to assist the designer in minimising cement stresses or other design objectives. Finally, some closing remarks are made to put current designs and design philosophies into perspective.

The Load-Transfer Mechanism

When a prosthetic stem is loaded it transfers the joint force to the bone. In the region of the prosthetic head, where the load is applied, the prosthesis alone carries the hip joint force. However, in the diaphyseal area distal to the prosthesis, the bone carries all the load. In between these regions, the load is transferred from the stem to the bone. How this is achieved is called the "load-transfer mechanism" [4]. Load-transfer is governed by stresses generated in the materials and at their interfaces. The likelihood of mechanical failure depends on the stress levels relative to the strength of the material considered. How the presence of a prosthesis affects

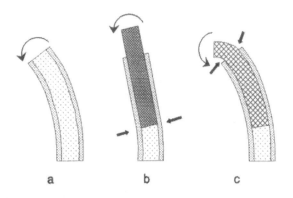

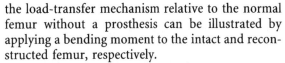

Fig. 3.1. **a** The "natural" bending deformation of a long bone. **b** Insertion of a relatively stiff prosthesis reduces the deformation around the prosthesis. Especially at the distal end of the prosthesis (arrows), the bone will move relative to the prosthesis as a result of the dynamic loading. **c** When a relatively flexible prosthesis is inserted, the deformation of the prosthesis is restrained, rather than the deformation of the bone. Especially at the proximal end (arrows), the prosthesis will move relative to the bone.

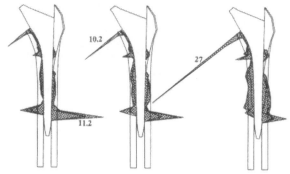

Fig. 3.2. Normal stresses at the bone implant interface for a CoCrMo, titanium, and "isoelastic" prosthesis. It is shown that with the flexibility of the stem the load-transfer can be governed to some extent. Flexible stems produce high stresses proximally, stiff stems produce high stresses distally. (Peak stresses are indicated in the figure.)

the load-transfer mechanism relative to the normal femur without a prosthesis can be illustrated by applying a bending moment to the intact and reconstructed femur, respectively.

Figure 3.1 schematically shows how a natural bone deforms under a bending load. When a stiff implant is inserted, bending will predominantly occur in the tip region. This causes high interface stresses between stem and bone in this area, and low stresses proximally. The opposite occurs if a stem that is more flexible than the bone is implanted. High proximal interface stresses are generated in this case.

Figure 3.2 shows the same phenomenon, but in a more realistic model. It shows the normal stresses at the interface for a very stiff cobalt–chromium stem, a relatively stiff titanium stem, and a relatively flexible "isoelastic" stem ("isoelastic" indicates that the stiffness of the prosthetic material is similar to that of bone itself). Proximal stresses are much higher for the flexible stem. Cemented stems usually have smaller diameters than uncemented ones, as a layer of cement is needed between the implant and bone. This makes the cemented stems more flexible than their canal-filling cementless counterparts, which results in a high amount of proximal load-transfer. For this reason, cemented stems are generally made of stiff materials such as cobalt-chromium alloys or stainless steel. A titanium cemented component would generally be too flexible, creating high interface and cement stresses at the proximal side of the reconstruction. This may explain the poor clinical results of the Capital Hip Prosthesis (3M

Health Care Ltd, Loughborough, UK) [5]. The femoral component of this system has a shape very similar to the Charnley prosthesis. Hence, the cross-sectional area is relatively small. The material of the Capital component is a titanium alloy whereas the Charnley prosthesis is made of stainless steel. In addition, the surface roughness of the Capital hip component is considerably higher compared to that of the Charnley. The most plausible failure scenario for the Capital hip stem is the creation of relatively high stresses in the proximal area due to the flexible metal component, thereby promoting stem–cement interface debonding and cement failure in these regions. The high surface roughness is likely to promote cement abrasion in this area.

Stem–Cement Interface Debonding and its Consequences for the Load-Transfer Mechanism

In retrieved specimens of cemented THRs, Jasty et al. [6] found areas of stem–cement interface failure long before clinical failure of the reconstruction was apparent. This led to the assertion: "The initiation of the failure process of cemented femoral THRs is now known, it is debonding of the stem–cement interface." [7] In our own retrieved material we also found that most of the stems were debonded from the cement mantle (Fig. 3.3).

That stems do debond from their cement mantles clinically can be detected by measuring the migration of the stem within the cement mantle. Migration

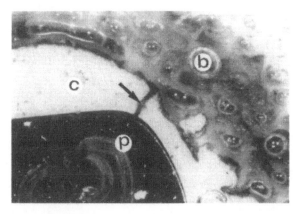

Fig. 3.3. A transverse section of a post-mortem retrieved specimen. "c" indicates cement; "p" prosthesis and "b" indicates bone. The stem has debonded from the cement mantle and a cement crack is created around the corner of the stem.

of the component within the cement mantle would mean, by definition, complete debonding of the stem–cement interface.

One of the most accurate and effective ways to assess this is the use of Roentgen stereophotogrammetric analysis (RSA). Most, if not all, RSA studies show prosthetic migration to some extent [e.g. 8–10] (Fig. 3.4).

Hence, there is substantial evidence that all stems sooner or later debond from their cement mantle and subsequently migrate. This already illustrates that it may be very difficult to prevent stem–cement debonding completely. It is important therefore to consider the possibility and consequences of stem–cement debonding in the prosthetic design process.

Before discussing this in more detail, we consider a simplified model consisting of a tapered metal stem inserted in a cement mantle (Fig. 3.5).

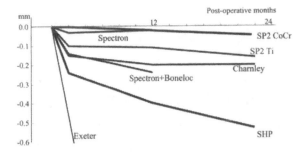

Fig. 3.4. Subsidence values of various total hip systems. Although one stem type seems to subside much more than the other, the results indicate that all stems subside and are therefore debonded from the cement mantle by definition (source: Nivbrant, Umea, Sweden; personal communication).

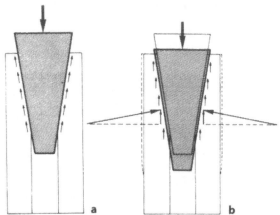

Fig. 3.5. Schematic representation of load transfer from a straight tapered cone pushed into a cylindrical counterpart. **a** With bonded interfaces, shear stress is developed to effectively equilibrate the compressive force applied. **b** At a smooth, press-fitted interface, equilibrium relies on the relatively small vertical component of compressive interface stress. The cone must subside to develop the required compressive stress values depending on the rigidity of the surrounding structure (reproduced from [10]).

The taper is axially loaded and the stem is assumed to be either bonded or debonded from the cement mantle. In both cases the force applied to the taper of the prosthesis has to be transferred to the cement at the interface. In the case of a debonded taper, load will primarily be transferred by means of compressive stresses. In addition some shear stresses can be generated, depending on the coefficient of friction between the two materials. For a bonded taper the shear stresses produced are generally much higher. The total sum of the axial components of the interface stresses is equal to the external load applied to the taper. When the taper is bonded, the shear stresses are important, because their components in an axial direction are relatively large. In the case of a debonded prosthesis, the axial components of the compressive stresses are small and the shear stresses are not high. Hence, high compressive stresses are necessary to compensate for the axial force applied to the taper. These high normal stresses can only be generated if the taper subsides in the surrounding material. A subsiding tapered stem produces high compressive stresses in a radial direction which are usually not very harmful because bone cement is relatively strong under compressive loads. However, a subsiding taper also generates relatively high hoop stresses in the circumferential direction. These are tensile stresses, as they expand the surrounding material. These stresses may cause material failure, with cracks oriented in radial and longitudinal directions [11, 12].

How and Where to Improve the Stem–Cement Interfacial Strength?

The interfacial strength can be enhanced by increasing the prosthetic surface roughness or the application of a cement precoated to the femoral stems [13–15]. Arroyo and Stark [13] investigated the effect of surface roughness on the shear strength of the stem–cement interface. An increase in strength from 0.8 to 10 MPa was found with increasing roughness from 1.6 to 7.7 μm. Crowninshield [14] found an 86-fold increase of shear strength when the surface finish was changed from 0.1 to 6.33 μm. Fatigue tests with specimens that were either precoated or uncoated showed that the precoated specimens had fatigue lives that were at least twice – and in some cases several orders of magnitude greater – that of the uncoated ones [15]. Knowing that improved interfacial strengths can be obtained, the question becomes in which areas the interface needs to be stronger. Retrieval studies show that stem–cement debonding starts at the tip and in the proximal regions [6]. Another way to demonstrate where the debonding process is initiated and how it progresses is to simulate the debonding process with finite element analysis (FEA). An example is shown in Fig. 3.6 [16].

The analyses confirm that the debonding process is initiated at the distal and lateral zones. The debonded zones extend progressively, until the whole interface is debonded. The stress component governing the debonding process was the shear stress, not the tensile stress. The latter remained very low during the whole debonding process. Hence, if

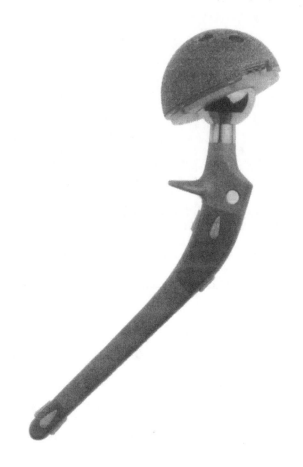

Fig. 3.7. The Centralign Hip System (Zimmer, Inc, Warsaw IN, USA) has a precoated area at the proximal and distal end. These are the areas where high interface stresses are expected. Debonding is postponed by increasing the stem–cement interfacial strength in these areas. Spacers are also applied at these locations to ensure adequate cement mantle thickness at these critical areas.

one wants to prevent stem–cement debonding it may worthwhile to strengthen the interface proximally and distally. This principle has been applied to the Centralign Hip System (Zimmer Inc, Warsaw, IN, USA) stem, which features a polymethylmethacrylate (PMMA) precoating at the proximal and distal surfaces (Fig. 3.7).

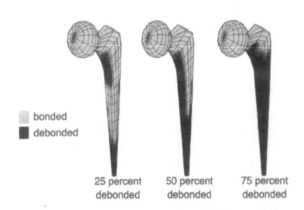

bonded
debonded

25 percent debonded   50 percent debonded   75 percent debonded

Fig. 3.6. The debonded sites at various stages in the debonding process as simulated with FEA. Debonding started at the distal and proximal aspects. These debonded sites expanded until the whole interface was loose (reproduced from [15]).

Reducing Cement Stresses Around a Debonded Prosthesis

An increase in interface friction will lead to increased interface shear stresses. Hence, high compressive interface stresses are no longer required to balance the external force, which then results in a stem that does not need to subside – and expand – within the cement mantle. This mechanism is shown in Fig. 3.8

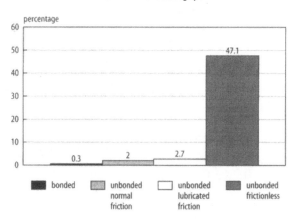

**Cement failure probability
after 10 million loading cycles**

percentage

bonded | unbonded normal friction | unbonded lubricated friction | unbonded frictionless

Fig. 3.8. The failure probabilities (FP) of the cement mantle after 10 million loading cycles. Stem–cement debonding increased the FP which was reduced again by increased friction at the stem–cement interface (reproduced from [16]).

where failure probabilities (FP) of the cement mantle are shown for an Exeter type stem.

FP is defined here as the percentage of cement volume stressed beyond the endurance limit at 10 million cycles [17]. A bonded stem produced the lowest failure probability, whilst a debonded stem produced a failure probability dependent on the coefficient of friction. The lower the coefficient of friction, the higher the failure probability of the cement mantle. It should be recognised that the case of a debonded stem with a zero coefficient of friction does not occur in reality but is merely an academic consideration to illustrate the extreme situation. It should be noted that even a highly polished stem does not behave as a frictionless interface, but creates a considerable amount of friction at the interface (coefficient of friction is about 0.25).

An increase of the friction coefficient is usually obtained by an increase in surface roughness. Although this will reduce stresses in the body of the cement at large, much higher stresses may occur locally, leading to cement abrasion. This can be illustrated with a simple experiment in which metal tapers with varying surface roughness values were inserted into cement mantles and then dynamically loaded [18]. All tapers debonded from the cement and gradually subsided into the cement mantles. Time-dependent subsidence was smaller with higher surface roughness values. Hence, the higher friction did indeed limit the subsidence. However, scanning electron microscopic (SEM) investigations showed that the damage in terms of abraded cement particles and cement cracks increased with higher surface roughness values (Fig. 3.9). Hence, ideally one would

like to have a higher coefficient of friction at the interface to reduce cement stresses while limiting the abrasive potential of the metal surface.

Another mechanism to limit the stress-elevating effects of stem–cement debonding is to increase the taper angle, which prohibits prosthetic migration and associated cement stress elevation. However, due to the fact that the stem has to fit within the femoral canal, the space to accommodate such a design feature is limited. One could also consider local elevations of taper angles, to prevent prosthetic migration and undesirable stress increases. It may then be more appropriate to use the term "prosthetic surface profiles" rather than tapers. In the extreme, a collar on a prosthesis could be viewed as a local taper with a taper angle of 90°.

The load-transfer mechanism is very sensitive to taper angles on the prosthetic surface. To illustrate this, consider a comparison of the mechanical behaviour between an Exeter stem (Howmedica International, Staines, UK) and an SHP stem (Biomet International, Swindon, UK) as simulated with finite element analysis [19]. The former stem is a double-tapered design with a very small taper angle (Fig. 3.10); the latter stem is an anatomically shaped prosthesis with a more pronounced taper angle (Fig. 3.11).

Upon loading, the Exeter stem subsided more into the cement mantle compared to the SHP stem. Subsidence values for the Exeter versus the SHP stem were: 220 versus 140 μm when no friction was assumed, and 32 versus 23 μm when realistic friction was assumed. As a consequence of the increased subsidence of the Exeter stem, the cement tensile stresses in the Exeter reconstruction were also higher compared to those encountered with the SHP stem. When stem–cement contact was assumed to be frictionless, the FP values were 47% for the Exeter and 10% for the SHP (Fig. 3.12).

The latter values are numbers to judge the differences in inherent stability. They do not give realistic estimates of actual cement failure probability, as frictionless contact does not exist. When both stems were assumed bonded to the cement, the FP-values were 0.3% for the Exeter and 0.2% for the SHP. For the unbonded analyses with realistic stem–cement friction, these increased to 1.8% in the Exeter, and to 0.3% for the SHP (Fig. 3.10). Hence, the larger taper angles (or more profiled shape) of the SHP stem reduced subsidence and adverse cement stress elevations. One should realise that although subsidence is limited by the increased taper angle, local stress elevations do occur in the area of the more pronounced taper. The extent of this stress elevation not only depends on the taper angle, but also on the frictional properties, the stiffness of the material and the overall shape of the component.

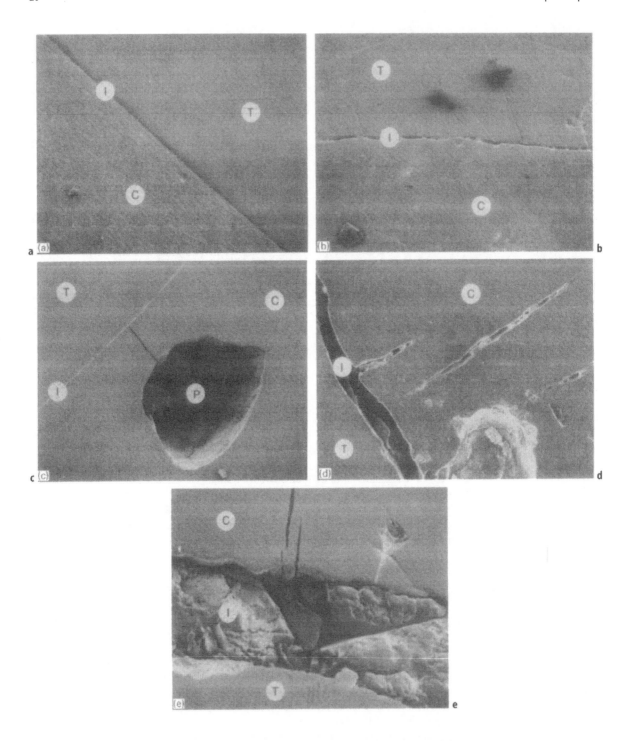

Fig. 3.9. A metal taper was inserted in a cement mantle and dynamically loaded. The roughness of the taper was either 0.033 μm (polished taper) or 9.96 μm (rough taper). The pictures show SEM micrographs of the cross sections of the taper and cement mantle composite; the markers represent 10 μm. ("C" indicates cement, "T" the taper, "I" the interface, and "P" a pore). **a** The interface in the unloaded (control) specimen of the polished taper could be identified as a line. **b** The interface in the unloaded (control) specimen of the rough taper had not fused completely, leaving gaps of up to about 10 μm. **c** In the loaded specimen with the polished taper, a crack was generated, associated with a big pore in the cement. **d** In the loaded specimen with the rough taper, a gap at the interface was formed and radial cracks were generated. **e** In the loaded specimen with the rough taper, acrylic cement particles were captured between the taper and the cement mantle (reproduced from [17]).

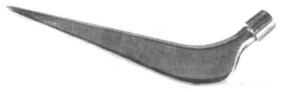

Fig. 3.10. The Exeter stem is straight tapered in the frontal plane, although it curves out medially towards the neck. Its anterior and posterior surface are virtually parallel. Its surface is polished.

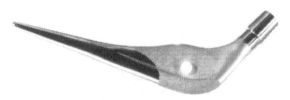

Fig. 3.11. The SHP stem is tapered proximally and distally, with a belly in the middle. It is curved in the sagittal plane. Its surface is grit blasted proximally and polished distally. Polymethylmethacrylate spacers are applied to guarantee adequate cement thickness.

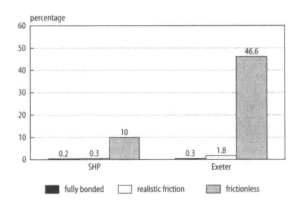

Fig. 3.12. Failure probability values for the Exeter and SHP stems, as determined with finite element analyses, for fully bonded stem–cement interfaces, unbonded with realistic friction (fully polished for the Exeter stem; proximally blasted and distally polished for the SHP stem) and for frictionless contact (reproduced from [18]).

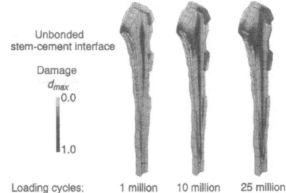

Fig. 3.13. The damaged sites in a part of the cement mantle of a debonded stem as predicted by a finite element simulation after 1, 10 and 25 million loading cycles of simulated loading. Cement damage primarily occurs at the corners of the stem resulting in radial and longitudinal cement cracks (reproduced from [22]).

As already mentioned, debonding and cement cracks are often found in retrieved postmortem specimens [6]. Endoscopic analysis of the cement mantle during revision THR surgery confirms that cement cracks do play a major role in the failure process of cemented THRs [20]. Koster et al. [20] reported that out of 23 revision cases studied, 21 showed either transverse or longitudinal cement cracks, which were often interconnected. Cracks were primarily found around the corners of the stems. This phenomenon can also be illustrated in finite element simulations where the accumulation of mechanical damage can be simulated, resulting in cracks in those locations where the stresses are maximal. An example is shown in Fig. 3.13, which demonstrates that for a debonded prosthesis cement failure will primarily occur around the corners of the metal component.

Hence, to maximise the mechanical endurance of the cement mantle, the radius of the stem contour should be as large as possible. In the extreme case this would lead to a stem with a circular cross-section. However, the stem would then probably have insufficient rotational stability, and might fail because of the anterior–posterior loading component present in most daily activities [21]. That rotational stability is a significant issue was demonstrated by a RSA study which showed that an implant with a rectangular cross-section exhibited virtually no internal rotation, whereas the component with a more circular cross-section produced significantly more rotation, sometimes progressing to early failure [9].

Using Computer Optimisation Techniques in Conjunction with Finite Element Analysis to Reduce Cement and Interface Stresses

Peak stresses within the reconstruction can be limited to some extent by adequate prosthetic shapes and materials. However, from the previous paragraphs it should be clear what the optimal shapes and materials are. Design goals can be incompatible (such as rounded corners with, at the same time, adequate rotational stability). Incompatible design goals need to be balanced to a certain extent [22]. To find an optimal balance, numerical optimisation routines can be used in conjunction with finite element methods. The optimisation method differs from the usual approach with FE analysis. Normally one has a particular design (shape and material properties) and determines the stress patterns within the structure under specified loads. In optimisation analyses this procedure is conceptually reversed, in that a desired stress pattern for a THR structure is specified, and the design characteristics by which it is realised are determined. The optimisation analysis is usually an iterative procedure (Fig. 3.14) and often starts with an initial design for which the stresses, strains, or other mechanical variables (e.g. strain-energy density, SED) are determined from the initial FE model.

If the stress distributions deviate from the desired ones, the shape or material characteristics of the design are adapted automatically in such a way that the stresses and strains are changed toward the specified values. This iterative process is repeated until the desired stress patterns are approximated as closely as possible, or within a specified range of error. The way in which the shape of the prosthesis is adapted in each iteration is determined by a search procedure that determines the search direction. Experience shows that it is an exception, rather than the rule, that the desired stress and strain distributions are realised precisely by the final design. One must be satisfied with a reasonable approximation of the desired stress and strain distributions. Fig. 3.15 shows an example of a numerical shape optimisation, starting with a conventional implant that

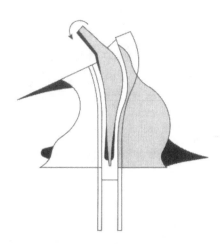

Fig. 3.15. Using optimisation routines in combination with the FEA method, the elastic energy in the cement at the cement–bone interface can be optimised. Dark: prior to optimisation; light: after optimisation (reproduced from [23]).

produces high stresses at the proximal and distal aspects and ending with a prosthetic shape that generates more evenly distributed stress patterns [23]. The same method can be applied to find the optimal material distribution within a femoral component of a certain shape that minimises the interface stresses [24].

Closing Remarks

We hope to have shed some light on the design considerations of cemented femoral components. At this moment, after more than three decades of research, it is somewhat frustrating to have to conclude that the ideal cemented femoral component has not yet been defined. This is due to the fact that the failure process is multifactorial. Probably the best way to approach this problem is to characterise the failure process as a collection of failure scenarios [22]. In this way it will be possible to ensure that a change of design (e.g. high prosthetic surface roughness) or material which is supposed to solve a particular problem (better bonding to cement) does not create other unexpected problems (considerable cement abrasion).

Currently, designs are based on a design philosophy rather than on proven scientific data. In this chapter three examples of stem designs have been discussed (Figs 3.7, 3.10, and 3.11) . The Centralign Hip System is based on the philosophy that a lasting stem–cement interfacial bond can be obtained and needs to be strengthened at those locations where high stresses are expected. Hence, it has a precoated

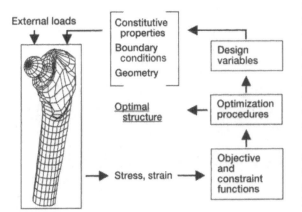

Fig. 3.14. A general scheme for iterative optimisation in combination with an FE-model (reproduced from [22]).

area proximally and distally. The current philosophy of the Exeter stem design is that stem–cement bonding cannot be obtained and therefore a stem needs a polished surface to minimise cement abrasion and a straight tapered design to accommodate subsidence. The philosophy of the SHP stem is based on minimised cement stresses (its geometry is based on NSO results). Initially the SHP stem was proximally and distally roughened, supporting the same design philosophy as the Centralign Hip System stem. But this was later changed to a polished distal aspect, where relatively high micromotions were expected, and a rough proximal part where the micromotions remain very small, even after complete stem–cement debonding [19]. These are just three examples of different philosophies and there are many others. The question which philosophy is the best cannot be answered yet; they probably all work for different reasons. However, perhaps a more relevant question would be what happens if the design philosophy fails. Is there a second line of defence incorporated in the design? An example of a stem with a fail-safe feature is the SHP. The surface roughness was chosen such that if debonding did occur, the consequences would be limited, as the micro-motions in the area where the rough surface is applied are expected to be very small. Whether this principle really works clinically has yet to be proven, as the SHP hip system is still in its early phase of clinical assessment.

Finally, we would like to suggest that newly designed hip systems be introduced to the orthopaedic marketplace stage by stage, using adequate preclinical tests to demonstrate that the design is safe relative to currently known failure scenarios, restricted clinical trials to prove that the design does not activate unexpected failure modes and post-marketing surveillance to ensure that the design works satisfactorily in the longer term [22, 25, 26].

References

1. Espehaug B, Havelin LI, Engesaeter LB, Vollset SE, Langeland N. Early revision among 12 179 hip prostheses. A comparison of 10 different brands reported to the Norwegian Arthroplasty Register, 1987–1993. Acta Orthop Scand 1996;67(2):113–114.
2. Malchau H, Herberts P, Ahnfelt L. Prognosis of total hip replacement in Sweden. Follow-up of 92 675 operations performed 1978–1990. Acta Orthop Scand 1993;64:497–506.
3. Paavolainen P, Hamalainen M, Mustonen H, Slatis P. Registration of arthroplasties in Finland. A nationwide prospective project. Acta Orthop Scand Suppl 1991; 241:27–30.
4. Huiskes R. Some fundamental aspects of human-joint replacement. Acta Orthop Scand Suppl 1980;185.
5. Massoud SN, Hunter JB, Holdsworth BJ, Wallace WA,

Juliusson R. Early femoral loosening in one design of cemented hip replacement. J Bone Joint Surg 1997; 79B:603–608.
6. Jasty M, Maloney WJ, Bragdon CR, O'Connor DO, Haire T, Harris WH (1991) The initiation of failure in cemented femoral components of hip arthroplasties. J Bone Joint Surg 73B:551–558.
7. Harris WH. Is it advantageous to strengthen the cement-metal interface and use a collar for cemented femoral components of total hip replacement? Clin Orthop 1992; 285:67–72.
8. Kärrholm J, Borssén B, Löwenhielm G, Snorrason F. Does early micromotion of femoral stem prostheses matter? J Bone Joint Surg 1994;76B:912–917.
9. Alfaro-Adrian J, Gill HS, Murray DW. The influence of prosthetic design on migration. A study of Charnley and Exeter THR with RSA. Transactions 45th Annual Meeting Orthopaedic Research Society, Anaheim, 1999.
10. Onsten I, Carlsson AS. Cemented versus uncemented socket in hip arthroplasty. A radiostereometric study of 60 randomized hips followed for 2 years. Acta Orthop Scand 1994;5(5): 517–521.
11. Huiskes R. The differing stress patterns of press-fit, ingrown and cemented femoral stems. Clin Orthop 1990;261:27–38.
12. Verdonschot N, Huiskes R. The effects of cement-stem debonding in THA on the long-term failure probability of cement. J Biomech 1997;30(8):795–802.
13. Arroyo NA, Stark CF. The effect of textures, surface finish and precoating on the strength of bone cement/stem interfaces. Proceedings 13th Society Biomaterials, New York, 1987: 218.
14. Crowninshield RD, Jennings JD, Laurent ML, Maloney WJ. Cemented femoral component surface finish mechanics. Clin Orthop 1998;355:90–102.
15. Raab S, Ahmed A, Provan JW. Thin film PMMA precoating for improved implant bone-cement fixation. J Biomed Mater Res 1981;16:679–704.
16. Verdonschot N, Huiskes R. Cement debonding process of total hip arthroplasty stems. Clin Orthop 1997;336:297–307.
17. Verdonschot N, Huiskes R. Mechanical effects of stem cement interface characteristics in total hip replacement. Clin Orthop 1996;329: 326–336.
18. Verdonschot N, Huiskes R. Surface roughness of debonded straight-tapered stems in cemented THA reduces subsidence but not cement damage. Biomaterials 1998;19:1773–1779.
19. Huiskes R, Verdonschot N, Nivbrandt B. Migration, stem shape, and surface finish in cemented total hip arthroplasty. Clin Orthop 1998;355:103–112.
20. Köster G, Willert HG, Buchhorn GH. Endoscopy of the femoral canal in revision arthroplasty of the hip. Arch Orthop Trauma Surg 1999 (submitted).
21. Bergmann G, Graichen F, Rohlmann A. Hip joint loading during walking and running, measured in two patients. J Biomech 1993;26: 969–990.
22. Huiskes R. Failed innovation in total hip replacement. Acta Orthop Scand 1993;64:699–716.
23. Huiskes R, Boeklagen R. Mathematical shape optimization of hip-prosthesis design. J Biomech 1989;22:793–804.
24. Kuiper JH, Huiskes R. Mathematical optimization of elastic properties: application to cementless hip stem design. J Biomech Eng 1997;119:166–174.
25. Malchau H. On the importance of stepwise introduction of new hip implant technology. PhD thesis, Göteborg University, Sweden, 1995.
26. Faro L.M., Huiskes R. Quality assurance of joint replacement. Legal regulation and medical judgement. Acta Orthop Scand Suppl 1992;250, 63:1–33.

Section II

Cement–Bone Interface

4. Histological Analysis of the Interface

H.G. Willert and G.H. Buchhorn

Introduction

Surgical implantation of endoprostheses provokes tissue reactions similar to those encountered at fracture healing. The bone which supports the implant is completely remodelled during and after this healing process. Thus the bone which receives the implant and which is responsible for primary stability is not the same bone which provides long-term support to the implant and which is responsible for secondary stability.

The interaction between the implant and the tissues of the implant bed ultimately decides the fate of an artificial joint replacement. This reaction falls into three overlapping phases [1, 2]:

1. *Immediate damage*: The initial phase comprises the insertion of the implant and the tissue damage caused by the procedure (during and immediately after implantation).
2. *Postoperative repair*: The phase of repair of the perioperative tissue damage (3 weeks to 2 years after implantation).
3. *Long-term stabilisation*: The phase of stabilisation in the permanent implant bed.

The three different aspects of the process embrace:

(a) the biology of healing and remodelling of the surrounding tissues,
(b) the biomechanics of adaptation of bone to the change in stress, and
(c) the chemical and physical effects of the implanted biomaterials upon the host tissues, such as irritation due to toxic components, mechanical instability, sepsis or accumulation of products of corrosion or wear [3].

The Initial Phase

Injury to the Tissues

Preparation of the implant bed causes considerable tissue damage. By reaming the medullary cavity we open the marrow spaces, ablate the bone marrow, crush and fracture parts of spongy and cortical bone and destroy the endosteal blood vessels (Fig. 4.1). As a result, a haematoma develops and the surrounding bone and bone marrow become necrotic (Fig. 4.2). This is very similar to the situation immediately after a fracture.

Load Transfer to Bony Structures

Painfree function is achieved with bone cement by penetration of the cement dough into the cavities of the bone. This provides initial stable fixation by anchoring the components to the bone. At this time load is transferred to the largest possible contact area with bone. In this phase there is no mobility at the interface that could interfere with healing [4].

It is necessary to understand the structures of the cement surface – as defined on retrieved components [5, 6] – in order to properly orientate the tissue bordering the cement. Based on the dimensional differences, these structures were divided into contours of 1st order (macroscopic range) and of 2nd order (microscopic range). First order contours are either even or papillary, and provide rough mechanical interdigitation with the prepared endosteal surface. The surface is irregular, wrinkled and wavy, corresponding with deep impressions into the former marrow-filled spaces between spongiosa and other

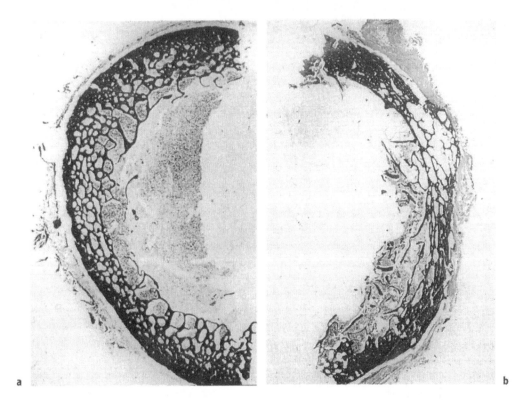

Fig. 4.1.   Bed of the cement implant **a** in the region of the greater trochanter, **b** in the shaft of an osteoporotic femur. Microphotograph from decalcified histological section, H&E stain, magnification **a** 5×, **b** 8×.

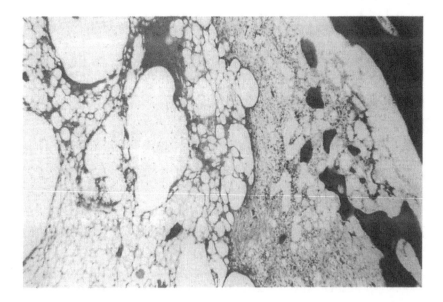

Fig. 4.2.   Initial phase: necrotic bone marrow and bone adjacent to the acrylic cement. Hyperaemic seams are bordering healthy bone. Microphotograph from decalcified histological section, H&E stain, magnification 40×.

bone protrusions. These surface structures are mainly to be found in the epiphyses and metaphyses of long bones and the spongiosa of the acetabulum. Much smoother, sometimes flat cement surfaces result from contact with cortical bone of the diaphyses of long bones or with subchondral sclerotic bone, e.g. of the acetabulum after reaming of the residual cartilage. The 2nd order surfaces are irregular, rough and open. Beads and contrast medium particles (ZrO_2 or $BaSO_4$ conglomerates) may protrude from the surface of the cement. Surfaces with strings of polymethylmethacrylate (PMMA) beads, connected by polymerised monomer matrix, are found in areas of high flow during cement insertion. All these surfaces give the impression of an open porous structure. Contact with flat bone surfaces under pressure flattens PMMA beads, which are then completely surrounded by the polymerised monomer matrix.

Response to Curing Cement

Necrosis occurs in cemented endoprostheses both as a result of preparation of the implant bed, and from the curing of the cement dough [2, 4]. Toxicity of leaching monomer has been discussed [7, 8]. Bone cement also generates heat during polymerisation. Both leaching monomer and heat may have a deleterious effect on the adjacent tissues. Necrosis has been found up to 3 mm from the cement surface [1, 9]. Despite extensive investigation, it is still not clear what proportion of necrosis in the direct vicinity of the cement is attributable to one or the other of the identified causes.

The Phase of Repair

Healing and Reorganisation of the Interface

Healing of tissue damage starts in the phase of repair (Fig. 4.3). Fibroblasts and capillaries grow from the adjacent intact tissues into the damaged areas, replacing the necrotic marrow by fibrovascular tissue (Fig. 4.3). The endosteal blood supply of bone, disturbed during surgery, is repaired by formation of a secondary medullary cavity near the interface [10, 11]. Within this fibrovascular tissue desmal bone is laid down very much like callus formation in fracture healing (Fig. 4.4). This implies that, during the phase of repair, new bone architecture can be formed where it has not previously existed. Even relatively wide clefts and defects can be filled and bridged by bone. Bone debris resulting from the reaming

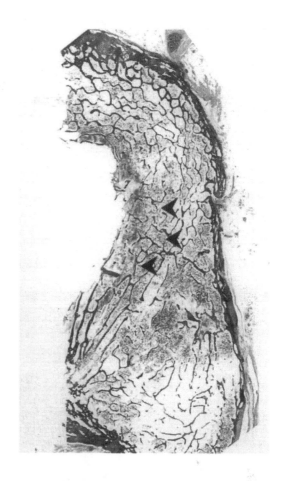

Fig. 4.3. Phase of repair: in the intertrochanteric region of the proximal femur the bone cement has dissolved out during embedding leaving an empty space ("c"). The bone trabeculae show the original regular orientation. Adjacent to the bone cement a zone of former perioperative tissue damage, now in the process of repair (arrow heads). Microphotograph from decalcified histological section, H&E Stain, magnification 3×.

procedure may also be incorporated in the new bone structures. In addition callus repairs fractured trabeculae [12] (Fig. 4.5). Good primary stability provided by implant fixation improves the preconditions for new bone formation, osseo-integration and secondary stability. Simultaneously, necrotic bone is removed by osteoclastic resorption (Figs 4.6 and 4.7). Bone trabeculae which are completely surrounded by bone cement will be resorbed and replaced by connective tissue [13].

Tissue sections at this early stage show how the second order cement structures are covered and penetrated by a latticed and rugged reticular tissue. The mulberry-shaped protrusions of PMMA pearls (cf. Fig. 4.12) are covered with macrophages and foreign body giant cells (Figs 4.4–4.6). Paraffin preparation technique removes the PMMA so that on the histological sections cells formerly in contact with the cement surface now surround empty spaces. Dense interdigitation results in conglomerates of

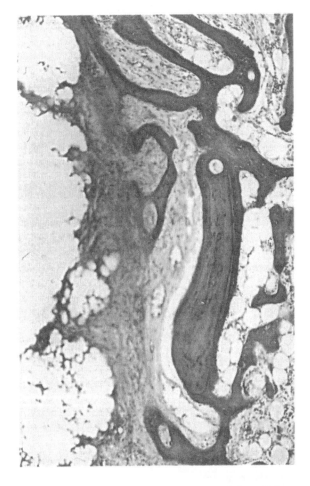

macrophages and foreign body giant cells, isolated within empty spaces and shaped according to the voids between cement beads. Where cement penetrated deeply into spongy bone, the trabeculae appear to be completely engulfed by PMMA.

New bone grows onto the surface of stable implants (e.g. filling in surface irregularities in the bone cement [2]). In 1987 Delling et al. reported only 20% direct contact between femur and bone cement surface, with even less for the acetabulum [14]. In 1992 Delling and Hahn calculated that only 2.7% of bone was in direct contact with cement in the whole bone–cement interface in the femur [13]. In the acetabulum Schmalzried et al. [15] and Bos et al. [16] found an almost complete separation between bone cement and bone.

The bone cement is lined with soft tissue between the areas of direct contact with bone. Ultimately, bone cement becomes almost continuously covered by giant cells [1, 2] (Figs 4.4–4.6).

Fig. 4.4. (Left)   Phase of repair: the acrylic cement (left) is covered with a thick fibrous tissue membrane (middle) that separates the spongious bone from the cement. Foreign body giant cells fill gaps between the cement pearls. Recently formed bone trabeculae seem to extend towards the cement implant. Microphotograph from decalcified histological section, H&E stain, magnification 100×.

Fig. 4.5. (Below)   Phase of repair: a layer of fibrous tissue rich in cells and of varying thickness covers the bone structures in opposition to the cement ("c"). Fractured and displaced trabeculae in the vicinity of the cement surface become reorganised. Osteoblasts lay down new bone (arrow heads). Microphotograph from decalcified histological section, H&E stain, magnification 100×.

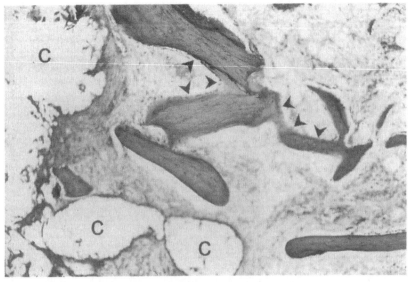

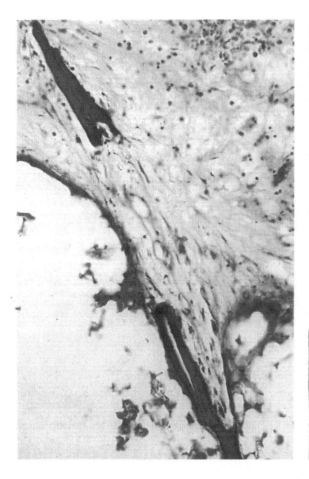

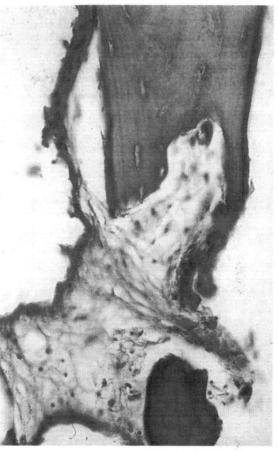

Fig. 4.6. Phase of repair: bone cement (in left half) is covered with thin layers of macrophages and foreign body giant cells. Spikes of pre-existent but necrotic bone become resorbed by osteoclasts and are replaced by a loose fibrous tissue. Microphotograph from decalcified histological section, H&E stain, magnification 250×.

Fig. 4.7. Phase of repair: a thin membrane of fibrous tissue separates a bone trabecula from the cement surface. Dead bone is resorbed by osteoclasts, the resulting space is filled with a fibrous tissue. Microphotograph from decalcified histological section, H&E stain, magnification 400×.

New Bony Structures and Their Adaptation to the Change in Load Transfer

Simultaneous with the repair of the perioperative damage, the bone adapts to the change in load transfer imposed by the implant according to Wolff's law [17]: In zones of decreased loading the bone mass decreases; this is associated with an expansion of the bone channels and marrow spaces. In zones of increased loading the bone mass maintains or increases its volume not only by filling in the marrow spaces but also by periosteal thickening of the cortex. The newly formed bone structures are orientated according to the new pattern of force transmission (Figs 4.1, 4.3 and 4.4).

There is a tendency to cover open marrow spaces, possibly in order to protect them against the flux of pressure caused by the intermittent loading of the implant. The cover can be provided by formation of cortical bone lamellae ("inner cortex"[10, 11]) or by dense fibrous tissue.

Direct attachment of bone to cement implants occurred preferentially at the convex surfaces of the polymer beads [13, 18]. Corresponding observations on non-cemented implants confirm this phenomenon as a principle of implant fixation [19–21]. It is not known whether this is biomechanically influenced or whether it is only a surface dependent phenomenon.

There is no doubt that the firm bond between bone and cement is based on intimate contact and "keying in" of the cement to fit the irregularities of the bone surface. However, the bony trabeculae which have to carry the cemented implant differ from those which were in contact with the cement at the time of implantation. Repair and remodelling completely change the bony bed and with consequent weakening of implant fixation. Even if bone extends right up to the cement by consoles or as a bony shell, the newly formed bone never exerts the same amount of pressure on the cement as at the moment of implantation [1, 9].

Tissue Response to Effects Inherent in the Implants

It is still not well understood why polymers like PMMA bone cement do not stimulate bone ongrowth onto their surface in the same manner as titanium. According to Boyan et al. [22], implant materials cause a biological response, which is obviously influenced by their chemical composition and surface texture. Several assumptions have been made regarding the factors affecting this response, e.g. dependence on the adsorption of serum proteins onto the material's surface or the release of mediators by cells in contact with the material. Moreover, implant materials probably interfere with the cascade of wound-healing and bone-growth factors and can affect osteoclastic activity; the morphology of matrix vesicle production is altered by the presence of implants and materials described as "bonding" promote matrix vesicle production, whereas those that are "non-bonding" do not [22]. It is still speculative to what extent surface geometry, surface chemistry or load transfer and micromotion (alone or in combination) are responsible for the various contact patterns identified: contact with macrophages and foreign body cells, non-calcified osteoid, bone and bone marrow, cartilage or with synovial like membranes.

The Phase of Stabilisation on the Permanent Implant Bed

Long-Term Structure of the Interface

In the phase of stabilisation, the interface between implant and bone consists of bony trabeculae, membranes of connective tissue of varying thickness, and of giant cells and macrophages which follow the contours of the conglomerated polymer beads [2, 6]. The function of these multinucleated giant cells is not yet known. Healthy haemopoietic and fat marrow is also found in the bone marrow spaces close to the implant.

However, seams of uncalcified osteoid are encountered in the vicinity of bone cement, even long after implantation (Figs 4.8 and 4.9). Charnley [10] described the calcified structures under the osteoid as older bone trabeculae laid down prior to cementation. Charnley [23], analysing decalcified tissue sections, described parts of these seams as "fibro-cartilage forming in fibrous tissue" which was said to be produced in response to mechanical contact with the cement. In a subsequent article [10], on the basis of non-decalcified sections, these "caps" on bone protrusions were also interpreted as being demineralized bone into which cement pearls had been pressed during load transmission. In undecalcified and trichrome-stained sections these osteoid seams and small beams are clearly separated by a

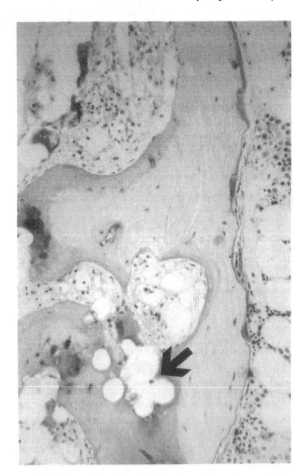

Fig. 4.8. Phase of stabilisation: part of the circumferentially orientated bone layer (inner cortex) in contact with bone cement (left margin) composed out of both bone anchors and fibrous tissue. The fibrous tissue is covered with foreign body giant cells whereas the bone anchors have caps of less mineralised bone and fibrocartilage. These caps engulf cement pearls in some places (arrow). Microphotograph from decalcified histological section, Giemsa stain, magnification 100×.

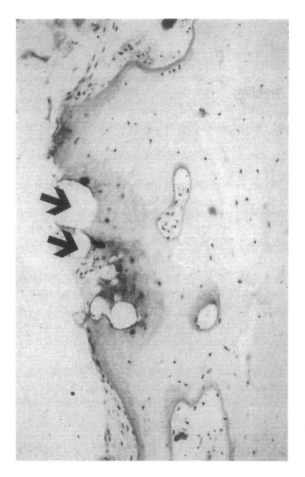

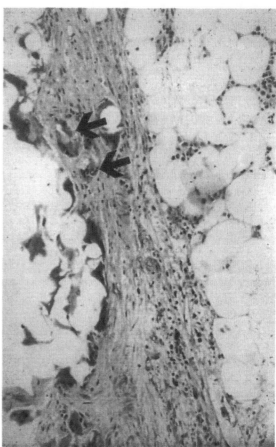

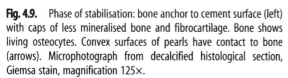

Fig. 4.9. Phase of stabilisation: bone anchor to cement surface (left) with caps of less mineralised bone and fibrocartilage. Bone shows living osteocytes. Convex surfaces of pearls have contact to bone (arrows). Microphotograph from decalcified histological section, Giemsa stain, magnification 125×.

Fig. 4.10. Phase of stabilisation: cement surface (left) separated from healthy fat marrow (right) by a fibrous tissue membrane containing macrophages and multinucleated giant cells. Direct contact to cement predominantly by foreign body giant cells extending deep into the irregularly formed open cement surface. Foreign body giant cells in the membrane store polyethylene wear and cement debris (arrows). Microphotograph from decalcified histological section, Giemsa stain, magnification 250×.

serrated line from the underlying calcified tissue. Lintner [24] and Delling et al. [14] interpreted this finding as a sign of disturbed mineralisation due to the toxic effects of the bone cement. According to Delling and Hahn [13] the proportion of bone showing these mineralisation defects is approximately 8.25% of the interface.

The connective tissue membrane formed during the phase of repair remains unchanged. It occurs between areas of direct bone contact, is of varying thickness and is sometimes very delicate. The giant cells remain permanently at the bone–cement surface, precisely outlining the contours of the bone cement's conglomerated polymer beads [2] (Fig. 4.10).

Remodelling of Bone

Implant fixation is finally established when the healing processes are complete. The fibrovascular tissue has then been entirely replaced by haemopoietic tissue, fat marrow and bone (Figs 4.8 and 4.10). Formation of completely new bony structures ceases, comparable to fracture healing, in which bony callus formation comes to an end after consolidation of the fracture. Then new bone will only be formed by apposition of osteoid lamellae by osteoblasts to the existing trabeculae. The creeping substitution of the original bone is achieved by resorption of bone anchors and apposition of lamellar bone to the remaining bone trabeculae. This occurs both during the remodelling sequence (which the implant-carrying bone is subjected to like any other bone) and in the course of bone adaptation to altered load transfer.

Endoprosthetic components may shield areas of bone against stress and change the direction of forces transmitted through the bone. The resulting atrophy presents as increased osteopenia. There are regions of the proximal femur which demonstrate bone loss of up to 60% after 12 years (e.g. Fig. 4.1a), while other areas remain unchanged. This process of bone loss also leads to a decrease in the number of anchoring bony trabeculae. Furthermore, during remodelling, the trabeculae seem to change direction from vertical to more parallel to the surface of the cement [1, 9] (Fig. 4.3). The creeping substitution of the original bone is achieved by osteoclastic resorption and subsequent apposition of lamellae to the remaining bony trabeculae by osteoblasts.

An increase in bone density of up to 25% [13] (with a spindle-shaped cortical thickening around or below the distal half of the femoral stem) signifies increased mechanical loading. Even around stable fixed endoprostheses apposition of osteoid on the trabeculae was observed infrequently on the side facing the cement, whereas seams of osteoblasts occurred more frequently on the side furthest from the cement [14].

Influence of Irritation Caused by Implants

The implant–bone-interface and the adjacent bone marrow proved to be highly reactive, especially to sepsis, mechanical instability permitting movement, products of corrosion, degradation products and wear from biomaterials. Common to all of these is the fact that they give rise to granulomata which stimulate osteoclastic bone resorption and lead to osteolysis. As bone resorption destroys the anchors of fixation, the implant loosens. This process is well documented in sepsis.

Grossly unstable implants permanently damage the tissue at the implant–bone interface and stimulate both bone resorption [25–27] and the formation of thick connective tissue membranes. The interface can however tolerate minimal movements between bone and cement in the sequence of weight-bearing and non-weight-bearing during walking. Such movements result from the different elastic properties of the rigid cement and the elastic bone (Figs 4.4 and 4.10). If these movements exceed the elastic capability of the tissue to deform at the bone–cement interface, rupture of the membrane occurs. We demonstrated haemorrhage and fibrin exudation

in numerous cases after long-term follow-up [9]. Fibrosis (after bleeding and exudation into the delicate tissue membranes of the interface) increases the thickness of the interface; sometimes these processes extend into the adjacent healthy bone marrow. Repair obviously results in a thicker contact membrane.

Charnley demonstrated areas within the interface where direct bone cement contact was maintained for 7 years of implant function. Though the extent was reduced in comparison to earlier stages of load transfer, he took this finding as proof "that no relative motion is taking place between cement and tissue" [10].

"Semistable" states with relatively smooth contact areas (as a result of minimal interdigitations between cement and bone) allow limited movement and are most likely responsible for the formation of "synovial like membranes" [28]. In these cases the connective tissue separating bone and bone marrow from the cement is covered with seams of cells that resemble synovial cells of the joint capsule (Fig. 4.11).

Slight micromovements under load bearing, due to a difference of elasticity in the contact zone, may also explain the differentiation of cells into cartilage. These areas show a structure histologically similar to direct bone–cement contact. However, in this situation contact is made by a relatively thin layer of cartilage which is interposed between the bone and the cement surface as a prolongation of the bone. These cartilage structures are often encountered where the second order structures are smooth (Fig. 4.9).

Any of these processes (atrophy, creeping substitution, adaptation to changed load transfer, overload-related tissue damage and cartilage transition) are said to produce radiolucent lines of varying thickness at the implant-bone interface due to loss of mineralised bone [29]. Maloney et al. [29] stated that these changes are a common finding in all long-functioning, cemented femoral components and are not necessarily a sign of loosening. In several of the specimens retrieved following aseptic loosening, however, they confirmed previous findings of soft tissue membranes formed in response to wear of the articulating surfaces of the joint and fatigue and fragmentation of the cement.

Abrasion, corrosion and degradation products are released from the articulation, the anchoring surfaces or modular interfaces, e.g. from the Morse taper. Abrasion is a mechanical process, and usually occurs as material wear at the articular surfaces or as a result of relative movements at the implant–bone interface. It generates microscopic and submicroscopic particles. Any material – metals, polymers,

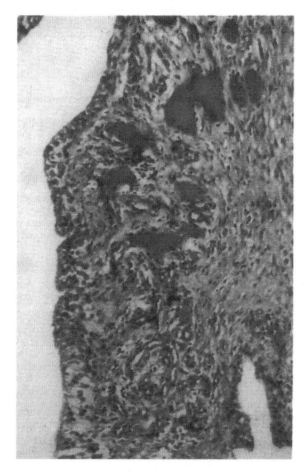

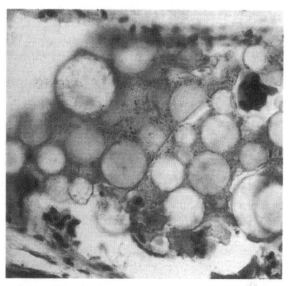

Fig. 4.12. Phase of stabilisation: acrylic bone cement surrounded by fibrous tissue. The pearls of the cement are cut at different heights, polymerised monomer matrix fills gaps in between the pearls. Macrophages, multinucleated giant cells, and fibrocytes cover the surfaces. Microphotograph from frozen section, Sudan stain, magnification 400×.

Fig. 4.11. Phase of stabilisation: soft tissue membrane with synovial like structure in contact with but not adherent to the cement surface. The membrane is lined by a multilayered synovial epithelium. Microphotograph from decalcified histological section, H&E, magnification 125×.

ceramics, carbon, etc. – is subject to wear; it is only the rate that differs.

Bone cement may fragment into small particles (Figs 4.10 and 4.12) due to propagating microfractures [31–33]. These induce a foreign body reaction with granuloma formation chiefly at the cement-bone interface, resulting in osteolysis. Factors which contribute to fragmentation of the bone cement are: increased load, irregularities and defects in the cement mantle, eccentric placement of the implant and direct contact between implant and bone resulting from a defective cement mantle (own unpublished results).

Particles released from the joint surfaces primarily induce a foreign body reaction in the capsule. Limited amounts of wear products can be stored in the capsule and eliminated by transport via the perivascular lymph spaces. Under these conditions

an "equilibrium" can be established, which allows almost undisturbed joint function in the long term [34, 35]. Entrapment of "third bodies" in the polyethylene articulating surfaces as well as changes such as fatigue or ageing of the material may increase particle production. Increased release of wear products dictates that tissues other than the joint capsule have to cope with the foreign material. In this state of "decompensation of storage and elimination" foreign body granulomas spread into the neighbouring tissues. The wear particles are transported away by three mechanisms:

1. via perivascular lymph spaces;
2. regional spread *per continuitatem* (by passive distribution within tissue structures);
3. dissemination of free floating particles via open communicating spaces.

The latter phenomenon was described for long transportation paths to the pole of a cemented acetabular component [15] and to areas distally in the femoral canal [33, 35 – 37] (Fig. 4.10).

Corrosion of implant alloys liberates soluble corrosion products as well as insoluble and sometimes particulate material [38, 39].

The ability of foreign body granulomas to destroy bone is prodigious. The richly cellular granulomatous tissue that stores foreign bodies expands not only into the plane of the implant/bone-interface, but also penetrates and infiltrates the bone canals and marrow spaces. Indeed, in some places, granulomatous tissues infiltrate the entire width of the cortical bone or perforate it completely.

Mechanically disturbed interfaces predispose to particle release. Movement between implant materials (cement/metal, cement/polyethylene) or implant material and bone causes deterioration of the surfaces, especially of the "weaker" material. Both may provoke bone-resorbing granulation tissue, which is responsible for osteolysis (radiologically observed as focal or seamlike areas of reduced mineralisation).

From the findings described above the following conclusions can be drawn. Apart from the traumatic procedure of implantation in the initial phase, the biocompatibility of the surface of the cement mantle determines the integration into bony structures during the phase of repair. Bridging of gaps and direct contact with bone is possible, though not as complete as, for example, with non-cemented titanium alloys [20,40]. The interface is sensitive to infection, trauma and any negative influences originating from the implants (i.e. particulate debris). These reactions often lead to loss of bone and aseptic loosening.

In the initial phase cemented anchorage of implants with cement is clearly superior to the anchorage of non-cemented devices. This is due to the extensive primary interdigitation of cement with bone and the ideal "form fit" between the cavity and the device. A high primary stability is consequently achieved.

In the phases of repair and stabilisation the bone of the implant bed adapts to the implant-specific load transfer. Given a perfect cementation technique and implantation the surrounding bone is able to support the cemented implant and compensate for inadequate load transfer over a long period of time. However, the stability achieved in the phase of implantation cannot increase, it can only be maintained.

Bone cement induces damage to the tissue during the initial phase and is not sufficiently biocompatible to encourage repair. The prevalence of macrophages and foreign body giant cells at the contact interface reflects the poor compatibility of the bone cement surface when compared with other materials (e.g. titanium). In the phase of stabilisation, significant changes in the material properties of the PMMA cement weaken the mechanical stability of the composite, thus endangering fixation and possibly leading to osteolysis.

References

1. Willert HG, Puls P. Die Reaktion des Knochens auf Knochenzement bei der Alloarthroplastik der Hüfte. Arch Orthop Unfall-Chir 1972;72:33–71.
2. Willert HG, Ludwig J, Semlitsch M. Reaction of bone to methacrylate after hip arthroplasty. A long-term gross, light microscopic, and scanning electron microscope study. J Bone Joint Surg 1974;56A:1368–1382.
3. Willert HG (1993) Endoprothesenverankerung mit oder ohne Zement? Z Orthop 113: 601–609.
4. Vernon-Roberts B, Freeman MAR. Morphological and analytical studies of the tissues adjacent to joint prostheses: Investigations into the uses of loosening of prostheses. In: Schaldach M, Hohmann, Thull R, Hein F (eds) Advances in artificial hip and knee joint technology. Springer Verlag, Belin-Heidelberg: New York, 1976; 148–186
5. Willert HG, Buchhorn GH, Zichner L, Müller K, Semlitsch M. Oberflächenstrukturen von Knochenzement. Z Orthop 1979;117:674–683.
6. Willert HG, Müller K, Semlitsch M. The morphology of polymethylmethacrylate (PMMA) bone cement surface structures and causes of their origin. Arch Orthop Traum Surg 1979;94:265–292.
7. Willert HG, Frech HA, Bechtel A. Measurements of the quantity of monomer leaching out of acrylic bone cement into the surrounding tissue during the process of polymerization. In: Gregor HP (ed) Biomedical applications of polymers. New York: Plenum Publishing Corp., 1974; 121–133 .
8. Hulliger L. Untersuchungen ueber die Wirkung von Kunstharzen (Palacos und Ostamer) in Gewebekulturen. Arch Orthop Traum Surg 1962;54:581–588.
9. Willert HG. Tissue reactions around joint implants and bone cement. In: Chapchal G (ed) Arthroplasty of the hip. Stuttgart: Georg Thieme Verlag, 1973; 11–21.
10. Charnley J. Low Friction Arthroplasty. Heidelberg, NewYork: Springer, 1979.
11. Malcolm AJ. Cemented and hydroxyapatite-coated hip implants – an autopsy retrieval study. In: Morrey BF (ed) Biological, material, and mechanical considerations of the joint replacement. New York: Raven Press,1993; 39–50.
12. Hahn M, Vogel M, Langendorff HU, Delling G. Mikrokallusformationen – Chronische Traumata des Skelettsystems als Stimulus des physiologischen Knochenumbaus. Hefte Unfallheilkunde 1991;220:523–524.
13. Delling G, Hahn M. Quantitative and qualitative analysis of the bone/cement-interface in relation to the structure of bone. Symposium Biomaterial "The implant / bone interface" 06-08.03.92, Göttingen, Germany, 1992.
14. Delling G, Kofeldt C, Engelbrecht E. Knochen- und Grenzschichtveränderungen nach Anwendung von Knochenzement – Langzeitbeobachtungen an humanem Biopsie-, Operations- und Atopsiematerial. In: Willert HG, Buchhorn GH (eds) Knochenzement. Bern: Huber Publishers, 1987; 163–171.
15. Schmalzried TP, Kwong LM, Jasty M et al. The mechanism of loosening of cemented acetabular components in total hip arthroplasty. Clin Orthop 1992;274:60–78.
16. Bos I, Lindner B, Seydel U et al. Untersuchungen ueber die Lockerungsursache bei zementierten Hueftgelenkendoprothesen Z Orthop 1990;128:73–82.
17. Wolff J. Das Gesetz der Transformation der Knochen. Berlin: Verlag Hirschwald, 1892.
18. Willert HG, Buchhorn GH. Osseointegration of cemented and noncemented implants in artificial hip replacement – Longterm findings in man. J Long-term Effects Med Impl 1998;9:113–130.

19. Willert HG, Lintner F. Morphologie des Implantatlagers bei zementierten und nichtzementierten Gelenkimplantaten. Langenbecks Arch Chir 1987;372:447–455.

20. Schenk RK, Wehrli U. Zur Reaktion des Knochens auf eine zementfreie SL-Femur-Revisionsprothese – Histologische Befunde an einem fuenfeinhalb Monate post operationem gewonnenen Autopsiepraeparat. Orthopaede 1989;18: 454–462.

21. Lintner F, Boehm G, Huber M. Zementfreie Schraubpfannen – Morphologische-mikroradiogaphische und morphometrische Untersuchungen zum Einbauverhalten. Med Orth Tech 1994;144: 233–237.

22. Boyan BD, Schwartz Z, Sela J et al. Biological implications – keynote address. In: Morrey BF(ed) Biological, material, and mechanical considerations of the joint replacement. New York: Raven Press, 1993; 27–34.

23. Charnley J. The reaction of bone to self-curing acrylic cement – a long-term histological study in man. J Bone Joint Surg 1970;52B:340–353.

24. Lintner F. Die Ossifikationsstörung an der Knochenzement – Knochengrenze. Acta Chir Austr Suppl 1983;48:3–17.

25. Charnley J. A biomechanical analysis of the use of cement to anchor the femoral head prosthesis. J Bone Joint Surg 1965;47B:354–363.

26. Scales JF. Acrylic bone cement: bond or plug. J Bone Joint Surg 1968;50B:689.

27. Perren SM, Huggler A, Russenberger M et al. Acta Orthop Scand Suppl 1969;125:19–28.

28. Goldring SR, Schiller AL, Roelke M, Rourke CM, O'Neill DA, Harris WH. The synovial-like membrane of the bone-cement interface in bone lysis. J Bone Joint Surg 1983;65-A:575–584.

29. Kwong LM, Jasty M, Mulroy RD, Maloney WJ, Bragdon C, Harris WH. The histology of the radioluent line. J Bone Joint Surg 1992;74B:67–73.

30. Maloney WJ, Schmalzried TP, Jasty M, Kwong LM, Harris WH. The cement interface: retrieval studies. In: Morrey BF (ed.) Biological, material, and mechanical considerations of the joint replacement. New York,:Raven Press, 1993; 51–70.

31. Kusy RP, Turner DT. Fractorgaphy of poly(methyl methacrylates). J Biomed Mater Res Symp 1975;6:89–98.

32. Lewis JL. The mechanical state of the bone-implant interface. In: Fitzgerald Jr R (ed) Non-cemented total hip arthroplasty. New York: Raven Press, 1988; 23–30.

33. Willert HG, Bertram H, Buchhorn G. Osteolysis in alloarthroplasty of the hip – the role of bone cement fragmentation. Clin Orthop Rel Res 1990;258:108–121.

34. Willert HG, Semlitsch M. Reactions of the articular capsule to wear products of artificial joint prostheses. J Biomed Mat Res 1977;11:157–164.

35. Willert HG, Buchhorn G, Buchhorn U, Semlitsch M. Tissue response to wear debris in artificial joints. In: Weinstein A, Gibbons D, Brown St, Ruff W (eds) Implant retrieval: material and biological analysis. US Department of Commerce, National Bureau of Standards, NBS SP 601, 1981; 239–267.

36. Anthony PP, Gie GA, Howie CR, Ling RSM. Localised endosteal bone lysis in relation to the femoral components of cemented total hip arthroplasties. J Bone Joint Surg 1990;72B: 971–979.

37. Schmalzried TP, Jasty M, Harris WH. Periprosthetic bone loss in total hip replacement: the role of polyethylene wear debris and the concept of the effective joint space. J Bone Joint Surg 1992;74A:849–863.

38. Willert HG, Buchhorn GH, Göbel D et al. Wear behaviour and histopathology of classic cemented metal on metal hip endoprostheses. Clin Orthop 1996;329S:160–186.

39. Willert HG, Brobäck LG, Buchhorn GH et al. Crevice corrosion of cemented titanium-alloy stems in total hip replacements. Clin Orthop 1996;333:51–75.

40. Böhm G, Lintner F, Brand G, Obenaus C, Klimann S. Morphometrische Befunde an einzelnen Titaniumschäften. In: Zweymueller K (ed) 10 Jahre Zweymueller – Hüftendoprothese. Bern: Verlag Hans Huber, 1990; 61–65.

5. Mechanical Analysis of the Interface

A. McCaskie

Introduction

During cemented hip replacement the surgeon creates a composite structure that comprises a central prosthesis, an interposed cement mantle and a surrounding layer of bone. Two interfaces are formed; the cement–bone interface and the cement–prosthesis interface and the long-term success of the new joint depends on the integrity of the interfaces. In considering the mechanical analysis of the cement–bone interface the importance of cementing technique must be emphasised.

The anatomical structures relevant to interface formation include the proximal femur which contains two types of bone, cortical and cancellous. The cortical bone has a compact structure and forms a hollow taper whereas the cancellous bone has an open structure with cavities between the bony elements (trabeculae). There are two important biological considerations; blood supply and bone marrow. The blood supply (derived from the nutrient artery system, periosteal supply and metaphyseal–epiphyseal supply) accounts for the bleeding surface encountered during arthroplasty. The trabecular spaces are filled with osteoprogenitor cells, haematological cells, water, fat and protein which can embolise during cementation causing physiological disturbance.

Fixation

Load applied to the prosthesis is transmitted through bone cement to the surrounding skeleton. To avoid high stress concentrations load transfer must take place over as large an area as possible. The trabeculated endosteal surface constitutes a large surface area but to achieve effective load transfer cement must penetrate the trabecular network and form a mechanically sound fixation with it, so-called microinterlock. As with an industrial composite the resulting mechanical properties depend upon the manufacturing process. In this case, the manufacturer is the operating surgeon and the manufacturing process is the cementing technique.

Charnley described a technique used in conjunction with trochanteric osteotomy [1]. Bone preparation involved curettage to remove loose cancellous debris and marrow, followed by packing of the canal. Cement was prepared in a mixing bowl by spatulation. The resulting ball of cement was kneaded (until no longer adherent to surgeon's glove) and inserted using a two thumb technique. Care was taken to both avoid admixture with blood and to impact cement into the proximal trabeculae. Further pressurisation was achieved by prosthesis insertion. The technique popularised by Charnley formed the basis for the evolution of "modern" [2] and "contemporary" [3] cementing techniques that aim to improve fixation [4].

Although it is one process, for the purposes of discussion, fixation can be considered using the following headings:

1. Surface preparation;
2. Cement type and mixing method;
3. Cement introduction and prosthetic implantation.

Surface Preparation

Any material that could be interposed between cement and bone (e.g. loose debris after reaming, bone marrow, and blood) should be removed. Various techniques exist and include:

1. Pulsed and continuous pressurised lavage;
2. Manual and power brushing;
3. Haemostatic agents;
4. Medullary packing;
5. Anaesthetic technique.

Blood forms both a static impediment as a clot and a dynamic obstruction as it flows under pressure in the opposite direction to cement. Hypotensive anaesthetic techniques, such as epidural anaesthesia, reduce the amount of blood at the interface and produce significant improvement in the radiological quality of the cement–bone interface [5]. Pressurised lavage (210 kPa) removes debris from the bone surface and produces significantly higher cement–bone interface shear strengths than those without lavage [6]. Comparisons between syringe, pressurised lavage and brushing suggest that the combination of pulsatile lavage, brushing and suction increases the interface strength fourfold [7]. Recent work evaluating blood contamination has aimed to "assess cementing technique in conditions more closely resembling those encountered in the operating theatre" [8]. Four insertion techniques; finger packing, restricted finger packing, Exeter, and low viscosity cement (LVC) (Zimmer, Warsaw, IN, USA) were used to create an interface in reamed ox bone either as a clean surface or with a thin film of blood applied. The interface shear strength was halved with the addition of blood when compared to the clean specimen. More recent work [9] using a bovine model has evaluated a comprehensive list of preparation techniques e.g. none versus 60 brush strokes, 10 brush strokes versus 60 brush strokes, 60 brush strokes versus lavage. There was an increase in the mean shear strength of the interface from 1.5 MPa to 9.9 MPa with brushing and up to 36.1 MPa with pressurised lavage. Also, using a bovine model, a significantly superior cement fixation (shear strength) was found using hydrogen peroxide as an irrigation fluid when compared with either normal saline or povidone iodine [10].

Canal restriction methods include a bone block [11] and a plastic or polymethylmethacrylate (PMMA) restrictor [12]. The theory of canal restriction is twofold. First, prosthetic insertion can push cement distally away from the area of fixation and into the marrow beyond. This can potentially lead to poor fixation [13], elevated intramedullary pressure [14] and embolisation of marrow [15–18]. Second, pressurisation of cement is facilitated by sound distal restriction against which pressure can be generated. A significant rise in intramedullary pressure has been demonstrated using a PMMA in situ plug with an associated increased cement penetration and cement–bone interface shear strength

[12]. A comparison between types of restrictor, using human femora, evaluated migration and ability to withstand and maintain a pressure of 400 kPa [19]. Polymeric restrictors were unable to maintain pressure and allowed distal leakage of cement. In addition, they were found to fragment on insertion. The PMMA restrictor was superior in terms of migration, leakage and ability to withstand pressure.

Cement Type and Mixing Method

Methods of void formation in cement include air entrapment during mixing, evaporation, thermal expansion and shrinkage. Hand mixing has the potential to trap air. Charnley said that he encouraged maximum aeration to counteract shrinkage and encourage monomer evaporation [20]. Despite this, there has been a trend to reduce porosity. This can be minimised by spatulating only long enough to mix the liquid and powder and then leaving the mixture to stand so allowing air bubbles to escape [21, 22].

Centrifugation of cement has produced a 54% increase in the mean ultimate tensile strength and a 136% increase in the fatigue life when compared to controls [23, 24]. In a study more comparable with the in vivo environment, the significant increase in fatigue life was maintained [25]. Centrifugation is most effective with reduced viscosity cements, with Simplex (Howmedica, London, UK) particularly responsive and original CMW 1 (DePuy CMW, UK) and Palacos® (Schering-Plough International, Kenilworth, NJ, USA) less so [26].

Vacuum mixing of cement can produce a 15–30% increase in flexural and compressive strength and modulus of elasticity [27]. Partial vacuum mixing by hand can reduce porosity from 7.2–9.4% to 0.1–0.8% with a 44% rise in uniaxial tension [28]. Further improvement is obtained when cement is mechanically mixed [29].

Porosity reduction is not favoured by all. There is some concern that with the reduction in voids the effect of shrinkage during polymerization might be exaggerated. This is particularly associated with large volumes of cement [30] but appears less relevant with volumes typical of a cement mantle [31, 32].

It has been suggested that initiation of cement polymerisation at the stem rather than the cement–bone interface would cause cement to shrink on to the stem rather than "shrink-away" from it [33]. Prostheses warmed to 44 °C before insertion were found to have dramatically reduced porosity at the stem–cement interface, a finding that may affect ultimate implant survival.

Only a proportion of the total time taken for a cement to polymerise is available to the surgeon for handling and cementation: the working time. The formulation can be altered to offer the surgeon a variety of cement viscosities in the working period. Original cements produced a dough ideal for thumb packing. The theoretical advantage of a low cement viscosity is that it will flow more easily into the trabeculae. Miller pioneered the use of LVC to achieve microinterlock [34]. However, LVC can be difficult to control at operation and must be used with precision; the cement must be inserted by instrument and the prosthesis should not be inserted immediately or cement will simply extrude. Reduced viscosity cements have been developed that utilise a viscosity between dough cements and LVC. These require sustained pressurisation to achieve and sustain microinterlock.

Cement Introduction and Prosthetic Implantation

In 1976, Markolf and Amstutz looked at the penetration and flow of cement [35] through drill holes in an aluminium disc (1, 2, or 3 mm diameter) with insertion at either 4 or 6.5 minutes after mixing. Penetration depth increased with increasing pore size, increasing applied pressure and early insertion. A second series, keeping the pore size constant (2 mm), varied the time over which pressure (23, 73, or 152 kPa) was applied. Similar changes with pressure and insertion times were found, but the majority of the penetration was achieved in the first 1–2 seconds of pressure application. A second study described the cement–bone interface pressure in four test conditions: early and late stem insertion, distal canal plugging, 1 or 2 mm mantles by rasp size and proximal seal during finger packing [36]. For late insertion, calcar pressure was higher in the unplugged group. The author explained that the existence of a distal vent allowed distal escape of cement and the prosthesis impacted the cement into the calcar more effectively. When plugged, cement extruded proximally and resisted stem insertion. Therefore, calcar pressure was lower. For early insertion, large pressures were recorded distally for plugged specimens (with low insertion force), whereas vented specimens allowed escape of cement and less pressure generation. Pressure was also recorded during finger packing of cement, prior to stem insertion. The values ranged from 130 kPa proximally to around 30 kPa distally.

Introducing cement from the proximal femur towards the distal end, as in finger packing, can trap blood and fat in the canal and create flaws in the cement mantle. Lamination of cement has been shown to significantly reduce tensile and shear strength [37]. Clearly, voids and debris will build up against the restrictor, and so venting of this space is required. Weber described the use of a suction vent and high viscosity cement, to avoid trabeculae being deeply penetrated by cement and the risk of necrosis and monomer toxicity [38].

Retrograde insertion is achieved by using a caulking gun with a long nozzle [39, 40]. The nozzle is placed against the restrictor and the gun withdrawn in a retrograde direction, filling the canal from distal to proximal. Retrograde filling has been shown to reduce laminations [21, 22, 41] and is an important feature of contemporary cementing technique [4].

Bleeding at the endosteal surface can cause disruption of the cement–bone interface [8, 9]. The endosteal bleeding pressure has been measured at 36 cmH$_2$O [42] and it has been suggested that, in a low viscous state, cement could actually be forced back out of trabeculae [43] or form laminations [44]. An experiment to simulate bleeding in a bovine model demonstrated a significant reduction in shear strength of the cement–bone interface in 50% of specimens using LVC [45]. Interestingly, there was no detrimental effect on cement penetration, suggesting that the fluid tracks alongside the cement rather than causing a bulk displacement of it. Sustained pressurisation maintains pressure on the cement until prosthetic insertion and aims to prevent medullary pressure falling below the bleeding pressure and to maximise flow into cancellous trabeculae. This can be achieved by digital pressure [12], mechanical impactor (solid or dynamic) [46] or proximal seal. The latter is used after canal filling when the nozzle is placed through the proximal seal and cut flush with it. The seal is placed hard against the femoral neck and held steady while more cement is triggered into the medullary cavity allowing sustained pressurisation [4].

The timing of prosthetic insertion is critical. When inserted too early cement will escape from the femur whereas if inserted too late excessive resistance will be encountered and the prosthesis will not seat properly. The pressure generated with insertion at the correct time may well be the most significant. With normal viscosity there is a shorter time interval between cement insertion and prosthesis insertion and therefore less time available for blood to contaminate the interface.

The application of pressure to an incompressible substance will cause it to flow through a porous structure. The fluid velocity is determined by the Darcy law [47]:

$$Q = A(k/\mu) \ (dP/dx)$$

where Q = volumetric flow rate; A = cross-sectional area; dP/dx = pressure gradient; μ = viscosity; k = constant.

It can be seen that flow/unit area (Q/A) is proportional to the pressure gradient and inversely proportional to the viscosity. Greater flow will be achieved by lowering the viscosity of the bone cement and increasing the pressure gradient applied to it and many papers have confirmed a link between pressure, penetration and shear strength. Halawa et al. demonstrated the benefit of increasing the pressure applied from 150 to 300 kPa [6] and Convery and Malcolm demonstrated that 700 kPa achieved 80% more penetration and 388% increase in shear strength [48].

The interface produced by a doughy cement compared with a low viscosity cement (170 kPa insertion pressure) has been compared in human tibial cancellous bone [49]. Experiments to test both tensile and shear properties demonstrated that pressurisation and careful preparation was associated with improved tensile and shear interface properties. Another study using a human cadaveric model evaluated the technique of retrograde filling with sustained pressurisation [50] and achieved complete filling of the canal. The majority of cement interdigitation was in the proximal third.

In 1983, Panjabi recognised that there were potential problems (e.g. embolisation) associated with high intrafemoral pressure, and suggested that a better understanding of the relationship between medullary pressure, penetration and the bone–cement composite was required [51]. Using canine femora, prepared as for hip replacement, cement was inserted using a custom syringe system that allowed the application of pressure for 15 seconds. On one side of a pair an insertion pressure of between 110–1230 kPa was used and on the other side the pressure was a constant 35 kPa. Using image analysis the absolute area of penetration and the relative area of penetration (percentage of available cancellous bone occupied by cement) was calculated. Relative penetration increased with insertion pressure. Penetration and pressure had a linear relationship between 250 and 550 kPa and the maximum penetration (90%) occurred with a pressure above 1200 kPa. The paper recommends 520 kPa as a pressure high enough to achieve adequate penetration of cement but sufficiently low to avoid complications. The following year the stiffness of the cement–bone composite was reported, using specimens prepared as before [52]. A steel rod was threaded into the centre of the cement and a bending force of 20 N was applied perpendicular to the long axis of the rod (less than that required to cause failure). A positive correlation between stiffness and penetration was demonstrated.

Askew evaluated the interrelationship between pressure, duration of application and viscosity [53]. Cement was pressurised into human cancellous bone at different pressures (8, 16, 39, 76, and 172 kPa) and for different time periods (5 or 30 seconds). Greater cement penetration and interface strength was produced with increasing pressure but there was no further improvement with longer application times. The failure patterns at the interface were divided into cement fracture, bone fracture, pullout and non-penetration. The trend was for cement fracture to occur when good penetration was achieved in strong bone whereas bone fracture failure occurred with weak bone. Pullout occurred at good penetration of moderate bone and the non-penetration failure mode is self explanatory. The recommended penetration level was 4 mm.

The pressure generated during stem insertion has been measured [54]. A cadaveric femur was prepared as for hip replacement and fitted with pressure transducers; proximal, middle and distal. After plugging, cement was mixed in a standardised way, inserted with a gun and digitally impacted. Large stems produced significantly higher pressure than small stems at all transducer positions. The pressure generated was maximal distally (758 kPa for large and 359 kPa for small) and much less at the proximal site (200 kPa for large and 131 kPa for small). With regard to shape, an arbitrary grouping called "rounded-rectangular" which included the Harris HD-2 and Charnley designs, achieved the highest pressure. It was concluded that the largest femoral stem that will allow a cement mantle should be used.

In 1988, Bean compared standard viscosity cement with a low viscosity cement in a closed system using human femora [55]. The applied pressure varied: 140, 280, 410 or 550 kPa and was applied for up to 10.3 minutes. A custom jig was used to drive cement into the specimen at the various pressures. Shear estimations were carried out at the bone–cement interface and through the cement itself. Penetration was also measured. Shear strength increased significantly with pressure but only up to 410 kPa. Further pressure did not improve this and there was no difference between cements in this respect. Cement penetration into cancellous trabeculae was complete in all cases regardless of cement or pressure applied. "Cortical" penetration was significantly greater with low viscosity and in this group the penetration rose with pressure. However, with standard viscosity cement penetration did not improve with pressure, in fact at 550 kPa penetration was less than at 280 kPa.

Using a sham replacement of the proximal femur in dogs, shear strength at the cement–bone interface was found to be linearly dependent upon depth of cement penetration [56]. Distal bone plugging and pressurised cement insertion brought about an 82% increase in shear strength and 74% increase in penetration with lower viscosity cement giving a further increase. Song et al. measured pressure continuously throughout cementation [57] demonstrating that the stem insertion produced the highest pressures. They suggested that prior impaction of the cement was probably unnecessary. Using human femora sections and servohydraulic tensile testing, they identified the extent of cement penetration into bone as the commonest determinant of interface failure [58]. There was a moderate positive relationship between the tensile strength of the cement–bone interface and the quantity of bone interdigitated.

Numerous variables influence the short- and long-term stability of the bone cement interface. Many of the experiments detailed above have qualitatively (or quantitatively) investigated one variable in vitro. Caution should be exercised in unquestioningly extrapolating these results to the complex environment – where many variables interact – in vivo.

Arthoplasty Simulation

Scientific innovation is required to reduce the incidence of failure of joint replacement. However, new cements have been associated with an increased rate of revision [59] while a high incidence of early aseptic loosening has been reported with certain new stems [60]. Innovation must be encouraged to allow progress but conversely it must also be controlled. A more cautious introduction of products has been proposed to improve the situation [61, 62]. The controlled introduction of technology should have pre-clinical and clinical elements. Preclinical testing, whereby a laboratory model attempts to simulate aspects of the clinical situation, can identify problems before clinical trials are undertaken. The accuracy and limitations of the simulation is the key to the usefulness of the data produced.

There is no consensus as to the best method of cementation and many techniques are currently practised [63–65]. Low loosening rates and excellent clinical results have been reported with both "modern" [3, 66, 67] and "early" techniques [68, 69]. Modern cementing techniques, e.g. retrograde filling, cement-gun, distal plug, and proximal seal used in conjunction with careful bone bed preparation using pulsatile lavage reduces the risk of revision [70]. Retrograde insertion of reduced viscosity cement and sustained pressurisation will tend to increase the degree of microinterlock but digital insertion of normal viscosity cement is still practised, presumably

because of both ease of use and lack of reason to change practice.

Over the last few years a programme of research has been undertaken to look in detail at cementation in the laboratory and develop a useful simulation. The arthroplasty model has the following features: human bone, paired testing, uses actual surgical techniques. The model assesses performance in terms of endosteal pressure generated, cement penetration into bone (using image analysis), and mechanical performance of the interfaces.

The simulation was validated in a study of pressurisation in hip replacement, comparing finger packing and retrograde insertion of cement [71]. This in vivo and in vitro study demonstrated higher peak and mean pressures with a gun technique, but less than some previously quoted in the literature [6, 48, 51]. The gun technique caused less physiological disturbance which may be explained by a combination of lavage and containment reducing the amount of material available for embolisation. The study observed much higher pressures when the stem was inserted, but noted that cement would be at a relatively higher viscosity and less inclined to flow.

Materials and Methods

Simulated Arthroplasty

Six pairs of human femora were obtained at postmortem [72]. Simulated arthroplasty was performed, in a safety cabinet, using a standard technique; neck osteotomy at an angle of 45° to the sagittal plane with calcar cut at the level of the vastus lateralis ridge and medullary reaming using tapered and curved reamers. A flanged 40 Charnley femoral stem (DePuy International, UK) was found to fit in all cases. The bone surface was prepared by removing loose debris, power brushing and pressurised lavage. A Hardinge cement restrictor (DePuy International, UK) was placed between 13.5 and 14 cm from the calcar. Before cementation, 3 ml of human blood were painted evenly over the endosteal surface to simulate the physical effects of bleeding (Bannister GC, personal communication 1993). The pressure effects of bleeding at the interface could not be simulated in this model.

For finger packing, normal viscosity cement (CMW 1, Depuy CMW, UK) was mixed as per manufacturer's instructions at 1 Hz, using a bowl and spatula. When the cement was no longer adherent to surgical gloves, the cement was digitally impacted into the femur. After a short period of sustained digital pressure the prosthesis was inserted. For the retrograde technique a reduced viscosity cement

(CMW 3, Depuy CMW, UK) was mixed as per manufacturer's instructions at 1 Hz, using a bowl and spatula. At 1 minute cement was poured into the gun barrel and at 2.25 minutes cement was introduced and pressurised. At 3.5–4 minutes the prosthesis was inserted.

The femora were sectioned perpendicular to the long axis by a microgrinding system using either a 0.2-mm diamond coated band saw (Exact, Germany) or a wafering saw (Isomet 2000, Buehler, UK). The first section was made through the calcar, and then at 7-mm intervals to produce 12 specimens per femur. Sections were numbered so that level 1 corresponded to the calcar and level 12 the tip of the stem (Fig. 5.1).

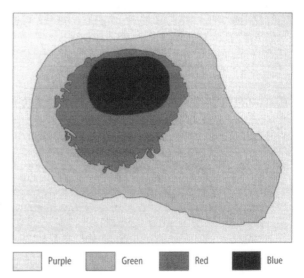

Purple   Green   Red   Blue

Fig. 5.3. All shades of grey have now been allocated a colour: blue for prosthesis, red for cement, green for bone, and purple for surround. This image is subjected to measurement of area and perimeter.

Image Analysis

All 144 specimens were evaluated by computerised image analysis (Omnimet 3, Beuhler, UK). The system used a video camera, frame grabber and computer software and hardware. The system was calibrated and an image of each specimen was "grabbed" by the computer (Fig. 5.2) and analysed by allocating a solid colour to the areas that corresponded to the prosthesis, cement and bone. This produced a four-colour image (Fig. 5.3). The area and perimeter of each block of colour were then determined, corresponding to the area of prosthesis, cement and bone. A single image was evaluated ten times to assess reproducibility. The results in Table 5.1 demonstrate the low standard deviation and high degree of reproducibility.

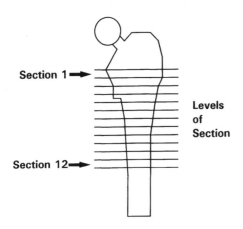

Fig. 5.1. Schematic diagram of the femoral specimen showing orientation and numbering of sections.

Mechanical Testing

Of the twelve sections per femur, levels 1, 4, 7, and 10 were tested mechanically. The testing rig, servohydraulic ram and 10 kN load cell were housed in a safety cabinet. The platform was fitted with a water

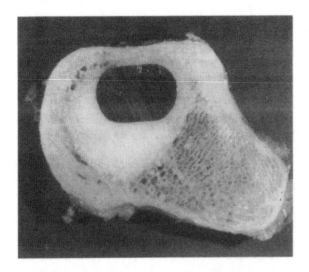

Fig. 5.2. Initial image of the femoral section in 256 shades of grey and stored digitally on screen: so-called "grabbed" image.

Table 5.1. The mean and standard deviations of the repeated estimations for a single image

Area of interest	Area/mm^2	Standard deviation
Prosthesis	147.8	0
Cement	243.7	0.2
Bone	1250.8	1.3

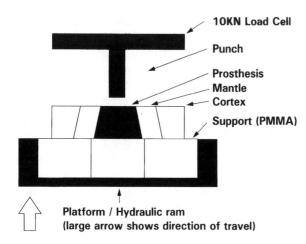

Fig. 5.4. Schematic diagram of the testing rig used to evaluate the cement–prosthesis interface.

bath to allow the specimens to be both hydrated and kept at body temperature during testing. The platform movement was detected by a linear voltage displacement transducer and force by the load cell.

To evaluate the cement-prosthesis interface, the cement was supported and load applied to the prosthesis (Fig. 5.4). Previously hydrated specimens were placed on the platform so that the surface originally nearest the tip was uppermost. Reverse pushout was then performed at a constant displacement rate of 4 mm/minute.

To evaluate the cement–bone interface, bone cement was moulded into the void left by the prosthesis and onto the upper mantle surface to act as a plunger, loading the specimen precisely at the cement–bone interface (Fig. 5.5). The test was performed in a similar way to that described above.

The data was non-parametric and so for each pair and at each level the difference between sides was

calculated. The differences were analysed by the Wilcoxon signed rank test, against a null hypothesis of no difference. A P value of less than 0.05 was considered significant.

Results

For image analysis the results were expressed as the percentage area of each specimen occupied by cement (Fig. 5.6). Except for the most proximal levels, the differences were in favour of the retrograde gun and differences were statistically significant at levels 6, 7, 8 and 11.

For the cement–prosthesis interface, the ultimate interface strength was calculated (Fig. 5.7). At all levels the gun technique achieved a larger value of

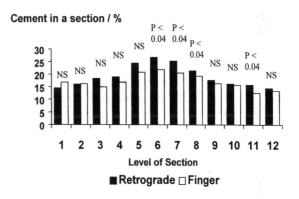

Fig. 5.6. Histogram showing the median values of cement area (expressed as a percentage of the whole) for each level. The significance of the difference is shown above.

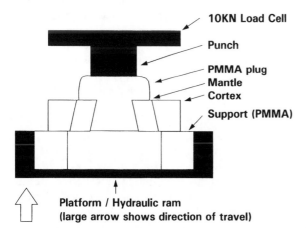

Fig. 5.5. Schematic diagram of the testing rig used to evaluate the cement–bone interface.

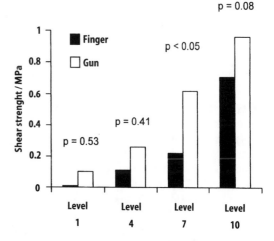

Fig. 5.7. Histogram showing the median values of ultimate shear strength, at each level, for the prosthesis–cement interface. The level of statistical significance of the difference is shown above the columns.

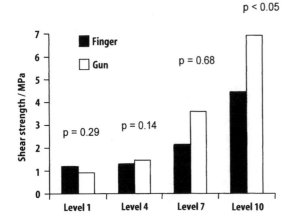

Fig. 5.8. Histogram showing the median values of ultimate shear strength, at each level, for the cement–bone interface. The level of statistical significance of the difference is shown above the columns.

shear strength than finger packing. At level 7 this was statistically significant and approached significance at level 10. Both techniques demonstrated a trend towards greater shear strength as the level of section moved distally.

For the cement–bone interface, again ultimate shear strength was calculated and the median values are shown (Fig. 5.8). Except for level 1 (calcar), the gun technique achieved a larger value of shear strength than finger packing and was statistically significant at level 10. Both techniques demonstrated a trend towards greater values as the level of section moved distally.

Discussion

Gun insertion produced significantly greater penetration at middle and distal levels. This broadly correlates with the pressure distribution observed during cement insertion rather than during prosthesis insertion [71]. This would support the hypothesis that the combination of relatively low interface pressure and reduced viscosity cement (i.e. during cement insertion) achieves more cement penetration than the combination of relatively high interface pressure and normal/high viscosity cement (i.e. during prosthesis insertion). This assumes that pressure is applied to the cement effectively by a careful surgical technique and that the pressure applied prevents blood disrupting the cement–bone interface. The model used in this experiment could not simulate the bleeding pressure and the results must be viewed accordingly. At distal levels the differences for penetration are not so marked as the pressure

differences, but at these levels the canal diameter is small and cancellous bone is sparse allowing only limited cement penetration irrespective of the applied pressures.

For prosthesis–cement interface strength, the differences were most notable at levels 7 and 10, with the gun technique appearing to produce a stronger interface. For both techniques the interface strength tended to increase along the length of the stem and this correlates with the pressures produced during prosthesis insertion, so that areas of high pressure are associated with high prosthesis–cement interface strength. The Charnley prosthesis has a "vaqua-sheen" finish with an undulating surface at a microscopic level. We hypothesise that there exists a "micromicrointerlock" between the prosthesis and cement and that the interface strength is determined by both cement and prosthesis insertion. The Charnley stem aims to achieve stability at the time of surgery and the bond between cement and prosthesis is enhanced by modern cementing. Debonding between cement and prosthesis may be a factor in loosening – although it cannot be equated with failure – and for this design may be resisted by modern cementation. However, the micromicrointerlock between prosthesis and cement may not occur with different stem designs and different surface finishes, e.g. highly polished. This would make an interesting future comparison. Interestingly, in a series of 17 early loosenings of a femoral stem with a surface coating designed to enhance the strength of the cement-prosthesis interface, it has been postulated that improving the bond at the cement–bone interface may transfer increased stress to the cement–bone interface and cause early failure at that interface [73].

The cement–bone interface showed no significant difference between the two techniques proximally, but at more distal levels the gun technique produced greater interface strength. The pattern of difference between techniques, minimal proximally and more marked distally, is similar to the pattern of differences observed for interface pressure (during cement insertion) and cement penetration. At proximal levels, for both techniques, cement was less able to penetrate to the corticocancellous junction. Examination of proximal level specimens after mechanical testing showed that failure had at times occurred through the trabeculae adjacent to the cement mantle. The interface strength would rely on the strength of the surrounding cancellous bone, and therefore be relatively independent of technique. This finding highlights the relevance of trabecular bone fatigue fracture in loosening and subsidence [74]. The situation differs distally, where cement more easily reaches the corticocancellous junction.

Both techniques created higher cement–bone interface strengths distally and with the gun technique the strength at level 10 was up to 10 times greater than at level 1. Concern over preferential distal interlock was already voiced by Charnley who wrote "one wonders whether to improve distal cement injection might not be counter-productive; it could be argued that we need 'controlled subsidence' of the distal half of the prosthesis stem to enable the cement in the upper end of the femur to maintain load-bearing contact" [1]. The pattern of lower cement–bone interface strength proximally and higher strengths distally is also observed when a proximal seal and sustained cement injection are used [75]. Early techniques, without a restrictor, may achieve this reverse gradient despite relatively low shear strengths in absolute terms and this could, in part, explain the clinical success of these early techniques [69]. It is suggested that modern techniques could improve proximal cement–bone interface strength further to improve proximal load transfer and prevent stress protection.

Further Developments

The sections produced by the above method have also been subjected to fatigue and creep assessment by altering the configuration of the servohydraulic test equipment [76]. The fatigue experiment was carried out on the submerged rig at body temperature and applied a force in the direction of physiological loading at 191 N at 4.66 Hz for over 900 cycles [77]. A pattern of initial slipping and then apparent stability (with slow subsidence) emerged on the curves of displacement against cycles. On four occasions the prosthesis was pushed out completely. In these cases there was an associated mantle defect that was not evident on conventional radiographic views of the femur taken before sectioning.

Using the above method, a further study to compare two "modern cementing techniques" has been performed [78]. The techniques used were a retrograde gun with either normal or reduced viscosity cements. The reduced-viscosity cement achieved significantly more penetration at proximal levels accompanied by a similar significant improvement in ultimate shear strength at the proximal area.

Many of these terms are comparative. Thus, the viscosity of the cement is influenced by the time of usage. It is hoped that the accuracy of the simulation can be improved and that combined with other mechanical tests a preclinical assessment can be developed.

Acknowledgements

The research could not have been completed without the efforts of others, in particular the head of department, Professor Paul Gregg. I would like to thank all of the following people who made contributions to the research programme: M.R. Barnes, A.R. Brown, P.J. Gregg, W.M. Harper, E. Lin, C. Morrison, M. Roberts, D. Rollings, and J.R. Thompson.

References

1. Charnley J. Low friction arthroplasty of the hip. Theory and practice. Berlin Heidelberg: Springer-Verlag, 1979.
2. Mulroy RD Jr, Harris WH. The effect of improved cementing techniques on component loosening in total hip replacement, an 11-year radiographical follow-up. J Bone Joint Surg 1990;72B:757–760.
3. Timperley AJ, Ling RSM, Jones PR. The effect of surgical technique on the quality of hip arthroplasty. J Bone Joint Surg 1992;74B:Suppl II:139.
4. Ling RSM. Cementing technique in the femur. Tech Orthop 1991;6(3):34–39.
5. Ranawat C, Beaver WB, Sharrock NE, Maynard MJ, Urquhart B, Schneider R. Effect of hypotensive epidural anaesthesia on acetabular cement–bone fixation in total hip arthroplasty. J Bone Joint Surg 1991;73B:779–782.
6. Halawa M, Lee AJC, Ling RSM, Vangala SS. The shear strength of trabecular bone from the femur, and some factors affecting the shear strength of the cement–bone interface. Arch Orthop Traumat Surg 1978;92:19–30.
7. Geiger JM, Greenwald AS. Comparison of surface preparation techniques at the bone cement interface. Orthop Trans 1980;4:266.
8. Bannister GC, Miles AW. The influence of cementing technique and blood on the strength of the cement–bone interface. Eng Med 1988;17(3):131–133.
9. Majkowski RS, Miles AW, Bannister GC, Perkins J, Taylor GJS. Bone surface preparation in cemented joint replacement. J Bone Joint Surg 1993;75B:459–463.
10. Howells RJ, Salmon JM, McCullough KM. The effect of irrigating solutions on the strength of the cement–bone interface. Aust NZ J Surg 1992;62:215–218.
11. Wroblewski BM, Van der Rijt A. Intramedullary cancellous bone block to improve femoral stem fixation in Charnley low-friction arthroplasty. J Bone Joint Surg 1984;66B:639–643.
12. Oh I, Carlson CE, Tomford WW, Harris WH. Improved fixation of the femoral component after total hip replacement using a methacrylate intramedullary plug. J Bone Joint Surg 1978;60A:608–613.
13. Wroblewski BM. Fractured stem in total hip replacement: a clinical review of 120 cases. Acta Orthop. Scand. 1982;53:279–284.
14. Tronzo RG, Kallos T, Wyche MQ. Elevation of intramedullary pressure when methylmethacrylate is inserted in total hip arthroplasty. J Bone Joint Surg 1974;56A:714–718.
15. Breed AL. Experimental production of vascular hypotension, and bone marrow and fat embolism with methylmethacrylate cement: traumatic hypertension of bone. Clin Orthop 1974;102:227–244.
16. Herndon JH, Bechtol CO, Crickenberger DP. Fat embolism during total hip replacement: a prospective study. J Bone Joint Surg 1974;56A:1350–1362.

17. Kallos T, Ennis JE, Gollan F, Davis JH. Intramedullary pressure and pulmonary embolism of femoral medullary contents in dogs during insertion of bone cement and a prosthesis. J Bone Joint Surg 1974;56A:1363–1367.

18. Harris NH, Miller AJ, Bourne R, Wilson S, Kind P. Experimental investigation of fat embolism after use of acrylic cement in orthopaedic surgery. J Bone Joint Surg 1975;57B:245–246.

19. Beim GM, Lavernia CJ, Convery FR. A comparison of intramedullary plugs used in total hip arthroplasty. Transactions of the 35th Annual Meeting of the Orthopaedic Research Society, 1989;369.

20. Charnley J. Acrylic cement in Orthopaedic surgery. Edinburgh: E & S Livingstone, 1970.

21. Lee AJC, Ling RSM, Wrighton JD. Some properties of polymethylmethacrylate with reference to its use in orthopaedic surgery. Clin Orthop 1973;95:281–287 .

22. Lee ACJ, Ling RSM, Vangala SS. Some clinically relevant variables affecting the behaviour of bone cement. Arch Orthop Traummat Surg 1978;92:1–18.

23. Burke DW, Gates EI, Harris WH. Centrifugation as a method of improving tensile and fatigue properties of acrylic bone cement. J Bone Joint Surg 1984;66A:1265–1273.

24. Burke DW, Gates EI, Harris WH. Improvement of tensile and fatigue properties of PMMA by centrifugation. Trans ORS 1984:128.

25. Davies JP, O'Conner DO, Burke DW, Jasty M, Harris WM. The effect of centrifugation on the fatigue life of bone cement in the presence of surface irregularities. Clin Orthop 1988;229:156–161.

26. Davies JP, Jasty M, O'Conner DO, Burke DW, Harrigan TP, Harris WH. The effect of centrifuging bone cement. J Bone Joint Surg 1989;71B: 39–42.

27. Lidgren L, Drar H, Moller J. Strength of polymethylmethacrylate increased by vacuum mixing. Acta Orthop Scand 1984;55:536–541.

28. Wixson RL, Lautenschlager EP, Novak MA. Vacuum mixing of acrylic bone cement. J Arthroplasty 1987;2:141–149.

29. Linden U, Gillquist J. Air inclusion in bone cement: Importance of the mixing technique. Clin Orthop 1989;247: 148–151.

30. Rimnac CL, Wright TM, McGill DL. The effect of centrifugation on the fracture properties of acrylic bone cements. J Bone Joint Surg 1986;68A:281–287.

31. Connelly TJ, Lautenschlager EP, Wixon RL. The role of porosity in the shrinkage of acrylic cement. Trans 13th Annual Society Biomaterials, 1987:114.

32. Jay JL, Noble PO, Lindahl LJ, Tullos HS. Porosity and the polymerisation shrinkage of acrylic bone cement. Trans 13th Annual Society Biomaterials, 1987:113

33. Bishop NE, Ferguson S, Tepic S. Porosity reduction in bone cement at the cement-stem interface. J Bone Joint Surg 1996;78B:349–356.

34. Miller J, Krause WR, Krug WH, Kelebay LC. Low viscosity cement. Orthop Trans 1981;5:352.

35. Markolf KL, Amstutz HC. Penetration and flow of acrylic bone cement. Clin Orthop 1976;121:99–102.

36. Markolf KL, Amstutz HC. In vitro measurement of bone-acrylic interface pressure during femoral component insertion. Clin Orthop 1976;121:60–66.

37. Gruen TA, Markolf KL, Amstutz HC. Effects of laminations and blood entrapment on the strength of acrylic bone cement. Clin Orthop 1976;119:250–255.

38. Weber BG. Pressurized cement fixation in total hip arthroplasty. Clin Orthop 1988;232:87–95.

39. Oh I, Harris WH (1982) A cement fixation system for total hip arthroplasty. Clin Orthop 164:221–229.

40. Lee AJC, Ling RSM. The Exeter system. Seminar and workshop handbook, 1983.

41. Lee ACJ, Ling RSM, Vangala SS. The mechanical strength of bone cements. J Med Eng Technol 1977;2:137–140.

42. Heys-Moore GH, Ling RSM. Current cementing techniques. In: Marti R (ed) Progress in cemented total hip surgery and revision: proceedings of a symposium held in Amsterdam. Amsterdam, Geneva, Hong Kong, Princeton, Tokyo: Excerpta Medica, 1982; 71.

43. Lee AJC, Ling RSM. Loosening. In Ling RSM (ed) Complications of total hip replacement. Edinburgh: Churchill-Livingstone, 1984;110–145.

44. Benjamin JB, Gie GA, Lee AJC, Ling RSM, Volz RG. Cementing techniques and the effect of bleeding. J Bone Joint Surg 1987;69B:620–624.

45. Majkowski RS, Bannister GC, Miles AW. The effect of bleeding on the cement-bone interface. Clin Orthop 1994;299:293–297.

46. Oh I, Bourne RB, Harris WH. The femoral cement compactor. J Bone Joint Surg 1983;65A:1335–1338.

47. Baeudoin AJ, Mihalko WM, Krause WR. Finite element modeling of polymethylmethacrylate flow through cancellous bone. J Biomechanics 1991;24(2):127–136.

48. Convery FR, Malcolm LL. Prosthetic fixation with controlled pressurized polymerisation of polymethylmethacrylate. Trans Orthop Res Soc 1980;4(2):205.

49. Krause WR, Krug W, Miller J. Strength of the cement-bone interface. Clin Orthop 1982;163:290–299.

50. Krause W, Bondy R, Miller JE. Sustained pressurization of acrylic cement in the proximal femur during arthroplasty. Trans Orthop Res Soc:1981;36.

51. Panjabi MM, Goel VK, Drinker H, Wong J, Kamire G, Walter SD. Effect of pressurization on methylmethacrylate-bone interdigitation: an in vitro study of canine femora. J Biomechanics 1983;16(7):473–480.

52. Panjabi M, Cimino W, Goel V, Drinker H. Enhancement of cement-bone composite by pressurization. Trans 30th ORS 1984;129.

53. Askew MJ, Steege JW, Lewis JL, Ranieri JR, Wixson RL. Effect of cement pressure and bone strength on polymethylmethacrylate fixation. J Orthop Res 1984;1:412–420.

54. Bourne RB, Oh I, Harris WH. Femoral cement pressurization during total hip replacement. The role of different femoral stems with reference to stem size and shape. Clin Orthop 1984;183:12–16.

55. Bean DJ, Hollis JM, Woo SLY, Convery FR. Sustained pressurization of polymethylmethacrylate: A comparison of low- and moderate- viscosity bone cements. J Orthop Res 1988;6:580–584.

56. Macdonald W, Swarts E, Beaver R. Penetration and shear strength of cement-bone interfaces in vivo. Clin Orthop 1993;286:283–288.

57. Song Y, Goodman S, Jaffe R. An in-vitro study of femoral intramedullary pressures during hip replacement using modern cement techniques. Clin Orthop 1994;302:297–304.

58. Mann KA, Ayers DC, Werner FW, Nicoletta RJ, Fortino MD. Tensile strength of the cement-bone interface depends on the amount of bone interdigitated with PMMA cement. J Biomechanics 1997;30(4):339–346.

59. Havelin LI, Espehaug B, Vollset SE, Engesaeter LB. The effect of the type of cement on early revision of Charnley total hip prosthesis. J Bone Joint Surg 1995;77A:1543–1550.

60. Massoud SN, Hunter JB, Holdsworth BJ, Wallace WA, Juliusson R. Early femoral loosening in one design of cemented total hip replacement. J Bone Joint Surg 1997; 79B:603–608 .

61. Murray DW, Carr AJ, Bulstrode CJ. Which primary total hip replacement? J Bone Joint Surg 1995;77B:520–527.

62. Malchau H. On the importance of stepwise introduction of new hip implant technology, Thesis, Goteborg, 1995.

63. Tillman RM. An improved femoral vent in cemented total hip arthroplasty. J Bone Joint Surg 1992;74B:Suppl II:140.

64. McCaskie AW, Gregg PJ. Femoral cementing technique: trends and future developments. J Bone Joint Surg 1994; 76B:176–177.

65. Hashemi-Nejad A, Birch NC, Goddard NJ. Current attitudes to cementing techniques in British hip surgery. Ann R Coll Surg Engl 1994;76:396–400.

66. Harris WH, McCarthy JC, O'Neill DA. Femoral component loosening using contemporary techniques of femoral cement fixation. J Bone Joint Surg 1982;64A:1063–1067.

67. Roberts DW, Poss R, Kelley K. Radiographic comparison of cementing techniques in total hip replacement. J Arthroplasty 1986;1:241–247.

68. Joshi AB, Porter ML, Trail IA, Hunt LP, Murphy JC, Hardinge K. Long-term results of Charnley low-friction arthroplasty in young patients. J Bone Joint Surg 1993; 75B:616–623.

69. Schulte KR, Callaghan JJ, Kelley SS, Johnston RC. The outcome of Charnley total hip arthroplasty with cement after a minimum twenty-year follow-up. The results of one surgeon. J Bone Joint Surg 1993;75A:961–975.

70. Malchau H, Herberts P. Prognosis of total hip replacement. Surgical and cementing technique in THR: a revision-risk study of 134 056 primary operations. Scientific Exhibition 63rd AAOS, 1996.

71. McCaskie AW, Barnes MR, Lin E, Harper WM, Gregg PJ. Cement pressurisation during hip replacement. J Bone Joint Surg 1997;79B:79–84.

72. McCaskie AW, Roberts M, Gregg PJ. Human tissue retrieval at post-mortem for musculoskeletal research. Br J Biomed Sci 1995;52:222–224.

73. Gardiner RC, Hozack WJ. Failure of the cement–bone interface. A consequence of strengthening the cement-prosthesis interface? J Bone Joint Surg 1994;76B:49–52.

74. Taylor M, Tanner KE. Fatigue failure of cancellous bone: a possible cause of implant migration and loosening. J Bone Joint Surg 1997;79B:181–182.

75. Ward AJ, Smith EJ, Barlow JW, Powell A, Halawa M, Learmonth ID. The in vitro measurement of cement–bone interface pressures and shear strengths in the femur: a comparison of two cementation methods. Hip Int 1995; 5:124–130.

76. McCaskie AW. Cemented femoral fixation. MD Thesis, University of Leicester, 1996; 236–247.

77. McCaskie AW, Brown A, Barnes M, Morrison M, Harper WM, Gregg PJ. Characterisation of a cement mantle defect leading to accelerated prosthetic subsidence. J Bone Joint Surg 1997;79B Suppl III:352–353.

78. Reading AD, McCaskie AW, Barnes M, Roberts M, Gregg PJ. Comparison of two modern femoral cementing techniques: in vitro study using cement–bone interface pressure and computerised image analysis. J Bone Joint Surg 1997;79B Suppl IV:468–469.

Section III

Modular Interface

6. Clinical Implications of Component Modularity in Total Hip Replacement

I.D. Learmonth

Modular components have certain distinct advantages and have been widely used at total hip replacement for almost two decades now. Modularity has provided the surgeon with the intraoperative flexibility to fine tune adjustments of limb length, offset, anteversion, head size, the requirement for and position of extended lip liners, etc. However, the levy for these benefits is the associated risk of fretting, corrosion, accelerated polyethylene wear, dissociation, etc.

It has been suggested that modularity results in cost saving, as it reduces the requirement for an extended inventory of different sizes. However, this apparent cost benefit is offset by the increased manufacturing costs generated by the tight tolerances required for these interfaces, and in the longer term by complications associated with modularity.

Chmell et al. [1] used data from their total joint registry to assess the influence of modularity on the outcome of total hip replacement. They noted that with each incremental increase in modularity there was an earlier and increased incidence of radiolucencies, osteolysis and aseptic loosening. It would therefore seem appropriate to analyse the benefits and risks of component modularity in clinic practice.

Acetabular Component

Polyethylene wear was identified as one of the main potential causes of failure of total hip replacement more than three decades ago. In 1970 Harris [2] developed a metal-backed acetabular component to allow replacement of the plastic bearing insert if wear was excessive. It was, however, not until the 1980s that the metal-backed acetabular components were modified to accommodate screw fixation, and provided with polyethylene inserts that would accept a wide range of head sizes (Fig. 6.1).

Advantages

Two-piece components allow screw fixation of the shell. While under-reaming and an interference press fit is currently the preferred method of fixation at primary hip arthroplasty, the availability of screw fixation is particularly useful at revision arthroplasty. If the polyethylene liner is worn or damaged, it can be selectively replaced at revision surgery. In addition, changing the insert permits the surgeon to change the size of the femoral head at isolated revision of the femoral component.

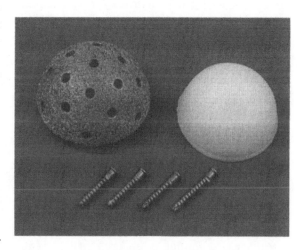

Fig. 6.1. A first generation modular cementless acetabular component – the HGP (Zimmer, Warsaw, IN, USA).

Extended lip liners can be dialled into the position providing optimum cover and stability determined at trial reduction. In difficult cases (spastic hemiplegia, paralysis, etc.) constrained liners can be used to enhance stability.

It should be noted that all discussions about modular acetabular components relate to cementless implants. Ritter et al. [3] reported that cemented metal-backed cups did not produce the predicted benefits, and their use has been largely discontinued.

Disadvantages

The use of a metal-backed shell inevitably means that the polyethylene thickness will be reduced. Bartel et al. [4] have shown that when the thickness of polyethylene falls below 6 mm the contact stress and amount of creep increase dramatically. This is particularly true with the relatively low surface contact area (and commensurate increase in surface stress) at articular interfaces in an artificial hip joint.

I believe that excessively thin polyethylene is the single most important cause of accelerated plastic wear in modular cementless acetabular components. Collier et al. [5] reviewed 111 acetabular explants, and noted that in some the polyethylene thickness was less than 3 mm. In addition, many of the large diameter cups that could have accommodated thick plastic instead had very thick metal walls and thin polyethylene inserts.

Learmonth et al. [6] compared the incidence of osteolysis in 98 Porous Coated Anatomic (PCA) total hip replacements (Howmedica, Rutherford, NJ) with 32-mm heads and 66 hips in which 26-mm heads were used. The mean follow-up was 7.5 years, and both groups were well matched for age, sex and primary diagnosis. No osteolysis was documented in the 26-mm head group. In contradistinction 24% of the hips in the 32-mm head group exhibited osteolysis of variable severity. Osteolysis was only encountered in those hips in which the outer diameter of the cup was 52 mm or less. Figure 6.2 shows the relative thickness of the polyethylene in PCA cups with varying outer diameters where the inner diameter was 32 mm.

Heck et al. [7], however, reported complete failure of the polyethylene in 172 of 60 115 metal-backed sockets (29 per 10 000). This compared favourably with complete polyethylene failure in 77 of 3219 all polyethylene cups (239 per 10 000). The reported acetabular dissociation rate was 15 per 10 000.

Madhavan et al. (European Hip Society presentation, Beaune, June 1998) described accelerated polyethylene wear in 14 of a cohort of 165 primary total hip replacements (THR) in whom a 32-mm head was used. Accelerated wear was arbitrarily defined as

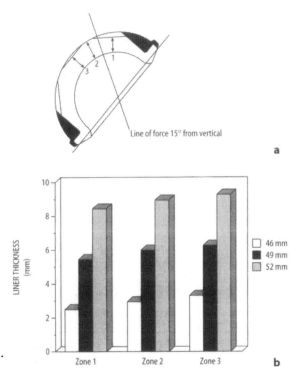

Fig. 6.2. **a** Schematic representation of a Porous Coated Anatomic (Howmedica, Rutherford, NJ) cup identifying three different areas in which polyethylene thickness was assessed. **b** Graphic representation of the thickness of the plastic liner when a 32-mm insert was combined with outer diameters of 46, 49 and 52 mm, respectively. The thickness in the three zones varies from 2.7 to 3.2 mm when the outer diameter is 46 mm.

being four times greater than normal. The thickness of the liner was less than 6 mm in all 14 patients. Table 6.1 shows the polyethylene thickness for different outer diameters of cups where a 32 mm head was used. It was of interest that these accelerated wear patterns were encountered between three and 5 years postoperatively (Fig. 6.3a, b).

There will always be relative motion between the polyethylene liner and the metal shell. Early locking mechanisms were often poor, and failure of the mechanism allowed the liner to spin in the shell with

Table 6.1   Shells and inserts in Harris Galante Porous 32–mm cups

Outer diameter	Shell thickness	Insert thickness
<48 mm	3.8 mm	<4.2 mm
50 mm	4.6 mm	4.4 mm
52 mm	4.6 mm	5.4 mm
54 mm	4.6 mm	6.4 mm
56 mm	4.6 mm	7.4 mm
58 mm	4.6 mm	8.4 mm

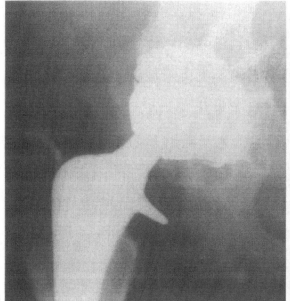
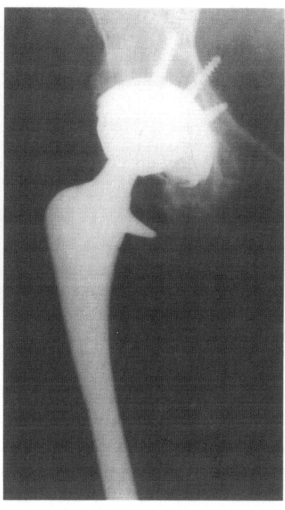

Fig. 6.3. a A 3-year postoperative radiograph of a cementless HGP prosthesis. The head is already slightly eccentric. **b** Five years postoperatively. Note the marked eccentricity of the femoral head, indicating complete wear of the polyethylene.

the generation of considerable plastic debris from the back face. In addition there have been several reports of component dissociation at the liner cup junction [8, 9,10]. We have seen this in 1 of over 1000 Harris Galante Porous (HGP) cups (Fig. 6.4).

Some degree of movement between the liner and the metal shell is inevitable. The more abrasive the interface the greater the amount of both metallic and polyethylene wear debris. Screw holes with sharp unpolished margins provide a potent source of abrasive wear. Huk et al. [11] identified sufficient early damage at this interface to suggest that the resultant wear debris would contribute to local macrophage mediated osteolysis.

Incongruency and gaps between the metal cup and liner will increase the stress on the polyethylene. Parsley [12] has shown that certain designs have gaps of up to 1.6 mm. Bono et al. [13] reported early failure with a cylindrical plastic liner and they ascribed this to a predisposition to rim loading. To

reduce this so-called "backside wear" one therefore requires congruency between the liner and the metal shell, a secure locking mechanism and a polished smooth acetabular shell surface. Chen et al. [14] reported a reduced debris production from highly polished acetabular shells, where the number of screw holes was limited and their edges were rounded off and polished. Bobyn et al. [15] also reported that a smoother finish diminished polyethylene debris from liner shell motion. However, Williams et al. [16] evaluated six modular acetabular systems and concluded that while surface polishing might reduce the amount of debris generated, the efficacy of the locking mechanism was the most significant factor that would prevent backside wear.

Lieberman et al. [17] identified three modes of damage (burnishing, punch-out and gouging) on the convex surface of polyethylene liners. Extrusion of polyethylene into the screw holes of metallic shells

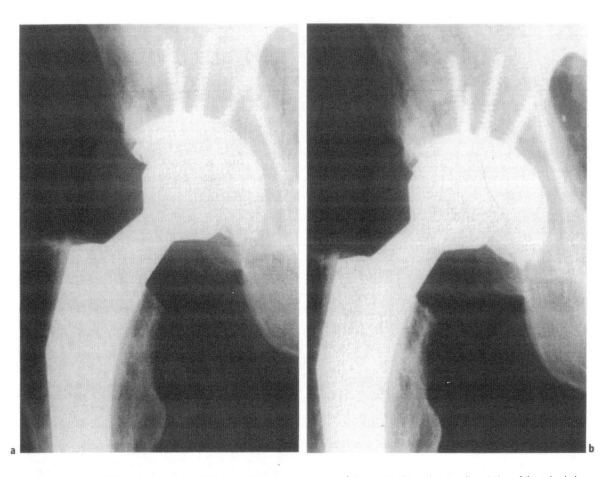

Fig. 6.4.   **a** A hybrid THR with a cementless HGP cup at 7 years postoperatively. **b** Six months later, showing dissociation of the polyethylene liner.

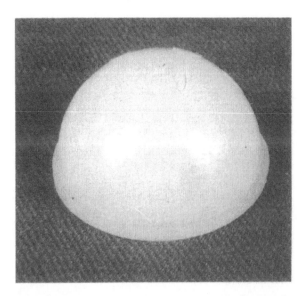

Fig. 6.5.   An explanted liner demonstrating visible crenellations on the outer surface as a result of the polyethylene deforming into the screw holes.

was universal in their in vitro analysis. We have also encountered this in explanted HGP cups, and the asperities on the polyethylene were almost exclusively encountered in the "weight-bearing" area of the cup (Fig. 6.5).

To prevent this shells are now available without holes or with a reduced number of holes. These are often "clustered" together in one quadrant of the cup, which can be rotated inferiorly – out of the weight bearing zone – if screw fixation is not required. In addition the holes in some shells can be filled before seating the liner.

Slight subsidence or settling of the cup may result in backing out and increased prominence of the screws. This results in deformation of the back surface of the liner and accelerated patterns of polyethylene wear.

Relative movement of the screw against the metal backing may result in fretting with the release of particulate metallic debris and focal osteolysis (Fig. 6.6). The screw hole also permits egress of polyethylene debris, which may itself provoke particle-mediated

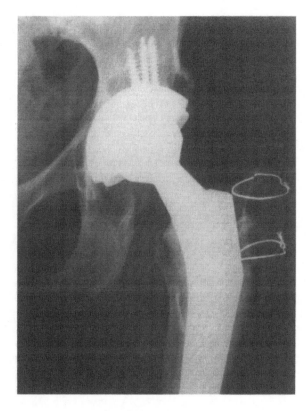

Fig. 6.6. Focal osteolysis superolateral to a well-fixed cup in an asymptomatic patient. This could be attributable to screw fretting or the escape of polyethylene from backside wear through a screw hole.

osteolysis. There are several reports of large cysts forming behind screw-fixed, metal-backed cups [11, 18]. However, in a prospective study of 130 HGP cups followed up for a minimum of 7 years, Learmonth et al. (European Hip Society presentation, Beaune, 1998) reported only two cases of focal periacetabular osteolysis related to screws.

Wasielewski et al. [19] have noted that hypotension and death have been reported from screw or drill penetration of the iliac vessels.

Summary

The production of debris depends on the contact stress and the amount and nature of the relative motion between mating surfaces when the joint is subjected to functional load and motion. The design should therefore: (i) provide a stable locking mechanism to minimise relative motion between the shell and liner; (ii) ensure congruency between the mating parts under load so as to optimise the stress distribution; (iii) avoid a rough finish or sharp edges around screw holes on the inner surface of the acetabular shell to limit the generation of debris;

(iv) decrease the number of screw holes (which decreases the area of contact between shell and liner, and so increases the stress in the plastic); (v) provide a cluster configuration (which can be turned out of the weight-bearing area); and (vi) a facility to close off unused holes.

Many of the problems and complications encountered with modularity of the acetabular component can be related to poor design features and can therefore be addressed by appropriate design modifications.

Femoral Component

Modularity of the femoral head clearly has apparent advantages. However, it also introduces certain disadvantages. It is therefore necessary to conduct a risk/benefit analysis to evaluate the rationale for current practice.

Advantages

Modular head/neck junctions (Fig. 6.7) have certain distinct advantages. They provide the surgeon with intraoperative versatility, allowing adjustments of leg length, offset, neck length (and thus stability), anteversion and fixation. This facility may be particularly valuable in developmental dysplasia and post-traumatic arthritis. It also supposedly reduces the inventory of implants that the theatre needs to stock for any given prosthesis.

Hozack et al. [20] reviewed a consecutive series of 100 primary cementless total hip arthroplasties (THA) where the neck length selected at trial reduction was compared with the final neck length chosen subsequent to the insertion of the femoral component. They

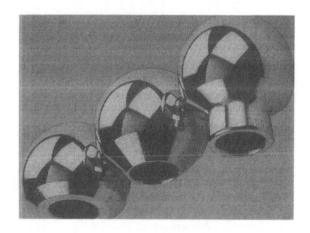

Fig. 6.7. Modular heads suitable for attachment to a Morse taper trunion.

reported that the final neck length differed from that at trial reduction in 19% of the hips. They felt that they were thus able to avoid limb length inequality or having to revise the femoral component.

There is little doubt that the seating of the definitive cemented stem sometimes differs from the trial, particularly when trial reduction is carried out with the broach in situ. In addition, McCarthy et al. [21] have noted that most cementless components have an "ideal seating level". Given this positional constraint, modular femoral heads provide the flexibility to restore limb length and joint stability.

A further advantage of modularity is that at revision of a loose acetabular component, where the femoral stem is well fixed, a damaged head can be exchanged. It should be remembered that a single scratch on the metal counter-face will produce an order of magnitude increase in polyethylene wear [22]. The ability to remove the femoral head also allows better exposure and visualisation of the acetabulum. In addition, if instability is identified at trial reduction following revision of the acetabulum, modularity provides a capability of obtaining stability with a longer neck or a larger head without having to revise the femoral component.

Titanium alloys are highly biocompatible and are widely used for implants that are inserted without cement. However, titanium alloys are relatively soft and scratch sensitive, and have been shown to be poor articular bearing surfaces which are associated with an increased rate of polyethylene wear. Modularity allows a combination of different metals to be used for the head and stem, and thus an optimisation of material properties.

Stem modularity beyond the head provides off the shelf customisation of calcar build-up and adjustment of neck version. This may be particularly useful in dysplastic hips, post-traumatic arthritis and following previous surgery to the proximal femur. Ries [23] has noted that many stems have modularity distally. This provides a unique opportunity to lengthen the stem by adding a distal attachment to cross the fracture site. Thus, a well-fixed proximal component can be left undisturbed while the stem extension provides appropriate intramedullary fixation.

Disadvantages

Rare instances of disassembly of modular heads (Fig. 6.8) have been reported. Pellici and Haas [24] described one such case, which occurred at attempted closed reduction of a dislocated hip. In a survey of 59 965 modular femoral heads, Heck et al. [7] reported the incidence of disassociation of the femoral head as 3 per 10 000.

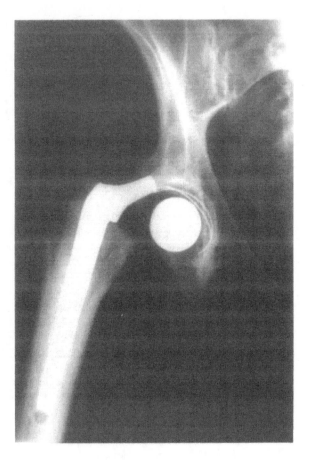

Fig. 6.8. Disassembly of a modular head.

The trunion itself often needs to be somewhat thicker than that required for a monobloc configuration to provide adequate strength. The head neck offset is thus reduced, with a consequent predisposition to early impingement. This will result in a reduced range of movement, while recurrent impingement will contribute to early loosening of the cup. A skirted head exacerbates these problems (Fig. 6.9a, b, c).

Krushell et al. [25] reported a reduced range of movement when a skirted modular head was used together with an extended liner. The longer-term implications of recurrent impingement were not considered. Chmell et al. [1] confirmed the increased risk of impingement and dislocation associated with a reduced head/neck ratio.

Harris [26] has suggested that all tapered junctions deteriorate with time. Fretting and corrosion at the modular interface are a cause of major concern. Collier et al. [27] have noted that if the metallurgy or design of the taper junction is suboptimal, it may provide an environment that predisposes to corrosion. They suggested that factors that

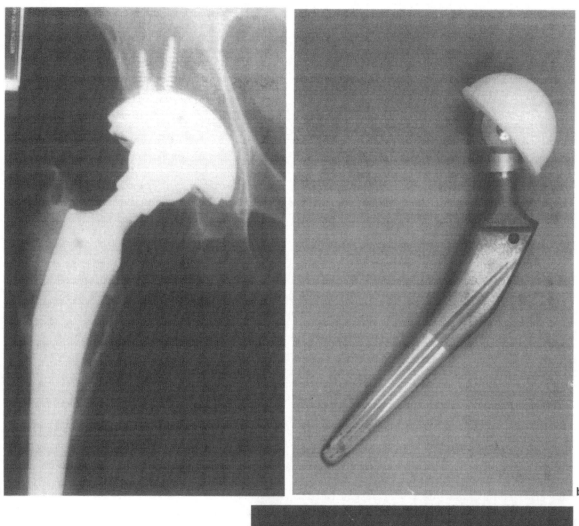

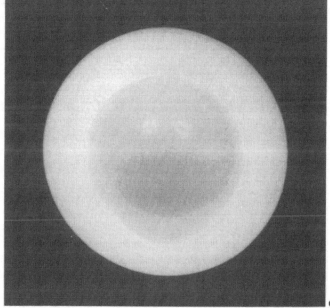

Fig. 6.9. **a** A skirted head as seen on a radiograph. **b** A skirted head shown impinging on the cup of an implant. **c** Focal damage on the rim of the plastic acetabular insert is clearly demonstrated.

contribute to corrosion include: (i) breakdown of the passive oxidation layer; (ii) heterogeneity of implant metals; and (iii) taper configuration. Crevice corrosion is encountered as a result of aqueous intrusion. In 1992 Collier et al. [28] reported on 139 retrieved modular femoral components. In the 91 in which the same alloy had been used for both head and stem there was no evidence of corrosion. However, definite corrosion was demonstrated in 25 of the 48 hips in which a cobalt-chrome head was applied to a titanium stem. They felt that this represented galvanically accelerated crevice corrosion.

This was supported by Lieberman et al. [29] who also reported corrosion with dissimilar metals but no corrosion where both stem and head were made of cobalt-chrome. Levine and Staehle [30] have shown that titanium alloy is susceptible to crevice corrosion and that a mixed alloy system would be likely to accelerate this process.

Cook et al. [31] observed detectable degrees of corrosion in 34.5% of mixed alloy stems and 9% of single alloy components that had been implanted for a mean of 25 months. They mechanically tested the modular head–neck interface to evaluate wear particle generation during cyclical loading. They showed that a significant number of wear particles were generated by all head–neck combinations. Approximately 2.5 million particles were generated during the first million cycles of loading, with 8 million particles being produced by 10 million cycles. All these particles had a size of less than 5 μm. Bobyn et al. [15] reported similar findings, and also reported that loaded tapers generated a large number of submicron particles. These metallic particles can, of course, represent a potent source of three-body wear.

Jasty et al. [32] found burnishing and scratching in 81% of uncemented and hybrid THA, and in 49% of cemented THA. Metallic debris arising from the modular taper junction was incriminated as the cause of this abrasive surface damage. Fretting damage and corrosion have also been encountered with ceramic heads, although much less frequently.

Mathiesen et al. [33] reported on macroscopic corrosion at the head–neck junction and tissue discoloration in four of nine retrieved femoral prostheses. The corrosion can be extensive (Fig. 6.10a, b) and is usually initiated low on the trunion, with intrusion of fluid.

Gilbert et al. [34] reported on severe corrosion culminating in the fracture beneath the head and neck taper.

Jacobs et al. [35] characterised the solid and soluble products of corrosion from the head and neck junction of modular femoral components. They identified particles of metal oxides, metal chlorides and calcium phosphate corrosion products on 10 different implants obtained from the manufacturers. They note that solid corrosion products may cause three-body accelerated wear of the polyethylene. In addition, phagocytosable particles of these corrosion products may stimulate macrophage mediated periprosthetic bone loss. Salvati et al. [36] have also described elevated synovial fluid levels of cobalt in patients with modular components.

Modular couplings distal to the femoral head are also associated with fretting wear, dissociation and an increased incidence of fatigue fracture. Huo et al. [37] reported burnishing of the femoral stem and evidence of metallosis within the medullary canal when a methylmethacrylate distal modular sleeve was used to maximise diaphyseal interference fit. It was postulated that this was due to fretting of the stem against the methylmethacrylate sleeve.

Chmell et al. [1] reviewed the data of their total joint registry over the past 25 years. They correlated results with the number of modular junctions present in their hip prostheses. They reported earlier radiolucencies, earlier aseptic loosening and earlier osteolysis (without aseptic loosening) with each incremental increase of modularity.

Summary

Fretting and corrosion at the head neck interface is clearly an important source of debris which may cause three-body wear and periprosthetic osteolysis. Severe corrosion may portend implant failure and fracture. It should be stressed that, although corrosion at the head/neck taper was widely reported, it was largely confined to a small number of implants. Nevertheless, most manufacturers have responded with concern, and have revised their specifications to provide better quality control of tighter taper tolerances. Care should be taken during the intraoperative assembly not to damage the modular surfaces or contaminate the modular interface with body fluids. Modular components from different manufacturers should not be mixed.

Head–neck modularity provides for an intraoperative flexibility that most surgeons would now be reluctant to forego. However, while possibly still desirable for highly polished double tapered stems and certain collarless cementless stems, it is probably not necessary for standard cemented THR, particularly if the stem has an easily identifiable endpoint. Modularity distal to the head and neck should probably be reserved for those cases not catered for by a comparable monolithic implant.

Fig. 6.10. **a** Extensive corrosion of a Morse taper (which had been thoroughly cleaned prior to taking the photograph). **b** The explanted femoral head shows extensive corrosion at the interface junction.

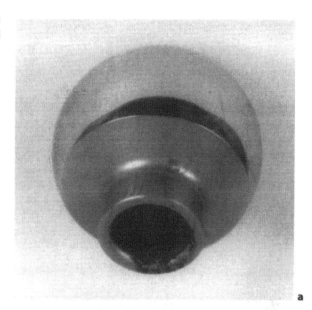

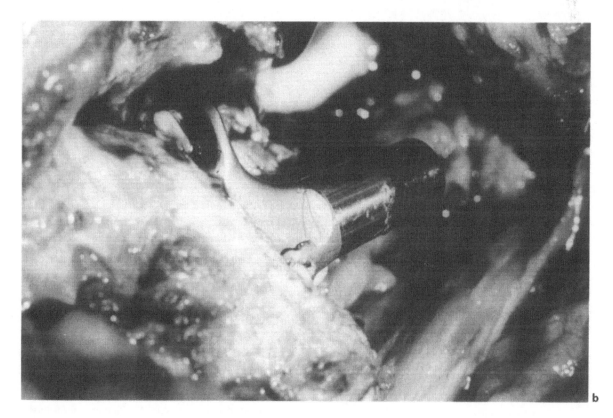

Conclusion

The Charnley Monobloc low friction arthroplasty (LFA) (and its immediate lineage) has been the most widely used implant over the past four decades. A wide selection of prostheses provided different offsets and different neck lengths. This gave a flexibility of choice at trial reduction, but a commitment following cementation. The excellent long-term results using the LFA are not marred by reports of significant limb length inequality (although it does happen – even with modularity!) or the necessity for early revision. The practical or technical case for modularity is thus less than persuasive. However, there is little doubt that modularity provides a reassuring intraoperative flexibility and versatility, which is of particular benefit at complex primary and revision hip arthroplasty.

The readily apparent advantages should not distract from the well-recognised disadvantages. Modularity in a hip replacement system can be either limited or extensive. The greater the modularity, the greater the degree of flexibility and the greater the degree of related complications. It does, therefore, seem appropriate to conduct a risk–benefit analysis from time to time to evaluate and clarify the rationale for current surgical practice. It is probable that in the future global economic constraints in health care will dictate that we tailor the prosthetic requirements to meet the patient demands.

References

1. Chmell MJ, Rispler D, Poss R. The impact of modularity in total hip arthroplasty. Clin Orthop 1995;319:77–84.
2. Harris WH. Modularity is unnecessary in primary femoral THA but has some advantage in primary acetabular THA. J Arthroplasty 1996;11(3):334–336.
3. Ritter MA, Keating EM, Faris PN, Brugo G. Metal-backed acetabular cups in total hip arthroplasty. J Bone Joint Surg 1990;72A:672–677.
4. Bartell DL, Bicknell VL, Wright TM. The effect of conformity, thickness and material on stresses in ultra-high molecular weight components for total joint replacement. J Bone Joint Surg 1986;68A:1041–1051.
5. Collier JP, Mayor MB, Jensen RE et al. Mechanisms of failure of modular prostheses. Clin Orthop 1992;285:129–139.
6. Learmonth ID, Hussell JG, Smith EJ. Inadequate polyethylene thickness and osteolysis in cementless hip arthroplasty. J Arthroplasty 1997;10 (3):305–309.
7. Heck DA, Partridge CM, Ruben JD, Lenzer WL, Lewis CG, Keating EM. Prosthetic component failures in total hip arthroplasty surgery. J Arthroplasty 1995;10 (5):575–580.
8. Bueche MJ, Herzenberg JE, Stubbs BT. Dissociation of a metal-backed polyethylene acetabular component. J Arthroplasty 1989;4(1):39–41.
9. Brien WW, Salvati EA, Betts F. Metal levels in cemented total hip arthroplasty: a comparison of well-fixed and loose implants. Clin Orthop 1992;276:66–74.
10. Kitzinger KJ, Delee JC, Evans JA. Dissassembly of a modular acetabular component of a total hip replacement arthroplasty. J Bone Joint Surg 1990;72A:621–623.
11. Huk OL, Bansal M, Betts F et al. Polyethylene and metal debris generated by non articulating surfaces of modular acetabular components. J Bone Joint Surg 1994;76B:568–574.
12. Parsley BS. Current concerns with modular metal-backed acetabular components. Proceedings of 59th Annual Meeting of the American Academy of Orthopaedic Surgeons, Washington, 1992; 83.
13. Bono JV, Sanford L, Toussaint JT. Severe polyethylene wear in total hip arthroplasty: observations from retrieved AML PLUS hip implants with an ACS polythylene liner. J Arthroplasty 1994;9:119–127.
14. Chen PC, Mead EH, Pinto JG, Colwell CW. Polyethylene wear debris in modular acetabular prostheses. Clin Orthop 1995;317:44–55.
15. Bobyn JD, Tanzer M, Krygier JJ, Dujoyne AR, Brooks CE. Concerns with modularity in total hip arthroplasty. Clin Orthop 1994;298:27–36.
16. Williams VG, Whiteside LA, White SE, McCarthy DS. Fixation of ultrahigh-molecular-weight polyethylene liners to metal-backed acetabular cups. J Arthroplasty 1997;12(1):25–31.
17. Lieberman JR, Kay RM, Hamlet WP, Park S-H, Kabo JM. Wear of polyethylene liner-metallic shell interface in modular acetabular components. J Arthroplasty 1996;11(5):602–608.
18. Tanzer M, Druker D, Jasty M, McDonald M, Harris WH. Revision of the acetabular component with an uncemented Harris Galante porous coated prosthesis. J Bone Joint Surg 1992;74A:987–994.
19. Wasielewski RC, Cooperstein LA, Kruger MP, Rubash HE. Acetabular anatomy and the transacetabular fixation of screws in total hip arthroplasty. J Bone Joint Surg 1990;72A:501–508.
20. Hozack WJ, Mesa JJ, Rothman RH. Head–neck modularity for total hip arthroplasty. J Arthroplasty 1996;11(4):397–399.
21. McCarthy JC, Bono JV, O'Donnell PJ. Custom and modular components in primary total hip replacement. Clin Orthop 1997;344:162–171.
22. Fisher J, Firkins P, Reeves EA, Hailey JL, Isaac GH. The influence of scratches to metallic counterfaces on the wear of ultra-high molecular weight polythylene. Proc Instn Mech Engr Part H 1996;209(H4):263–204.
23. Ries MD. Intra-operative modular stem lengthening to treat peri-prosthetic femur fractures. J Arthroplasty 1996;11(2):204–205.
24. Pellici PM, Haas SB. Disassembly of a modular femoral component during closed reduction of the dislocated femoral component. J Bone Joint Surg 1990;72A:619–620.
25. Krushell RJ, Burke DW, Harris WH. Elevated-rim acetabular components: effect on range of motion and stability in total hip arthroplasty. J Arthroplasty 1991;6:S53–58.
26. Harris WH. A new total hip implant. Clin Orthop 1971;81:105–113.
27. Collier JP, Mayor MB, Williams IR, Suprenant VA, Suprenant HP, Currier BH. The tradeoffs associated with modular hip prostheses Clin Orthop 1995;311:91–101.
28. Collier JP, Suprenant VA, Jensen RE, Mayor MB, Suprenant HP. Corrosion between the components of modular femoral hip prostheses. J Bone Joint Surg 1992;74B:511–517.
29. Lieberman JR, Rimmol CM, Garvin KL, Klein RW, Salvati EA. An analysis of the head-neck taper interface in retrieved hip prostheses. Clin Orthop 1994;300:162–187.
30. Levine DL, Staehle RW, Crevice corrosion in orthopaedic implant materials. J Biomed Mater Res 1977;11:553–561.
31. Cook SD, Barrack RL, Baffes GC et al. Wear and corrosion of modular interfaces in total hip replacements. Clin Orthop 1994;298:80–88.
32. Jasty M, Bragdon CR, Lee K, Hanson, A, Harris WH. Surface damage to cobalt-chrome femoral head prostheses. J Bone Joint Surg 1994;76B:73–77.
33. Mathiesen EB, Lindgren IU, Blomgren GGA, Reinholt FP. Corrosion of modular hip prostheses. J Bone Joint Surg 1991;73B:569–575.
34. Gilbert JL, Buckley CA, Jacobs W et al. Intergranular corrosion fatigue failure of cobalt alloy femoral stems : a fatigue analysis of two implants. J Bone Joint Surg 1994;76B:568–574.
35. Jacobs JJ, Urban RM, Gilbert JL et al. Local and distance products from modularity. Clin Orthop 1995;319:94–105.
36. Salvati EA, Lieberman JR, Huk OL, Evans BG. Complications of femoral and acetabular modularity. Clin Orthop 1995;319:85–93.
37. Huo MH, Fye MA, Martin RP, Zatorski LE, Keggi KJ. Unsatisfactory results of a first-generation modular femoral stem implanted without cement. J Arthroplasty 1997;12(5):490–496.

Section IV

Component–Bone Interface

7. Component Bone Interface in Cementless Hip Arthroplasty

J.D.J. Eldridge and I.D. Learmonth

Cemented total hip replacement is one of the most successful orthopaedic procedures, with reliable relief of pain and restoration of function. Long-term results have improved with modern cementation techniques resulting in the use of total hip arthroplasty in an increasingly young patient population. Despite reported stress survival rates of up to 98% at 20 years in young patients [1] other series report higher implant loosening rates [2–4]. Direct contact between cement and bone can occur but is rare, the usual interface being a fibrohistiocytic membrane described by Fornasier et al. [5] who also describe an inevitable loosening cascade at the cement–bone interface. Other factors implicated in the loosening of cemented prostheses include mechanical degradation of the acrylic bone cement with time [6, 7], impairment of mechanical strength of cement by contaminants [8], compromise of the host tissue by monomer leakage [9], and thermal injury to the bone during polymerisation [10], although this is disputed [11]. In addition, while cement is tolerated in bulk, it is known that particulate cement is ingested by and activates inflammatory cells, thus mediating osteolysis. These observations have stimulated interest in the development of a direct biological bond between prosthesis and bone using cementless fixation.

Principles of Cementless Fixation

The aim of cementless hip arthroplasty is to achieve a durable and lasting biological fixation of prosthesis to bone. In general, bone reacts to the presence of prosthetic implants in one of two ways. More commonly it forms a soft tissue membrane of either fibrous tissue or highly organised fibrocartilage. However, under certain conditions the bone integrates the prosthesis with a secure osseous bond. This reaction has been termed osseo-integration, implying direct contact between prosthesis and living bone with no interposed membrane (Fig 7.1).

This osseo-integrated interface will have much higher interfacial strength and stiffness than the fibrous interface [12, 13]. Some authors [14] believe a fibrous tissue layer can be effective in distributing stresses from prosthesis to bone while preventing proximal stress protection osteopenia [15]. There is, however, no reason to believe that this periprosthetic membrane will be any less prone to the loosening cascade than its equivalent in cemented arthroplasty. It is therefore now generally accepted that osseo-integration of at least part of the prosthesis is the goal of cementless arthroplasty, with the potential for permanent implant fixation. Maistrelli et al. [16] introduced the concept of functional osseo-integration. In combined histomorphometric and biomechanical analyses of hydroxyapatite (HA)-coated stems they

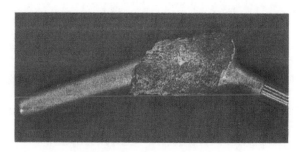

Fig. 7.1. An explanted PCA stem showing considerable bone ingrowth into the proximal porous coating.

noted two distinct types of HA bone interface. Type A was a thin, isolated bone plate formed on the coating and type B a bone plate buttressed by trabeculae radiating out to the cortex. Interface type B alone provided adequate implant support on pushout testing. Thus, bone ingrowth alone does not necessarily imply a successful outcome.

Biology of Cementless Fixation

Bone is one of the few tissues of the body that can repair without scar tissue formation. This repair process occurs in three phases. In the inflammatory phase there is haematoma formation followed by an acute inflammatory response. The reparative phase follows with invasion of the haematoma by fibrovascular tissue. Any necrotic bone is removed by osteoclasts and stem cells from the endosteum and periosteum differentiate into osteoblasts or chondroblasts depending on the microenvironment. Fibrocartilagenous callus fills the gap and stabilises the bone ends before being replaced with woven bone by endochondral or intramembranous ossification [17]. Under optimal conditions of stability and bone to bone contact primary or direct bone healing can occur [18]. Finally, in the remodelling phase functionally orientated lamellar bone replaces the woven bone. The process of bone ingrowth into a porous coated implant has been compared with bone repair and direct bone ingrowth has been shown to occur in stable press fit porous-coated implants [19]. If a gap of greater than 1 mm exists then endochondral ossification will be required.

The eventual outcome following a fracture may be either union through direct bone healing or endochondral ossification or non-union. The interfragmentary strain theory [20] hypothesises that high strains will result in fibrous tissue formation and low strains in chondral tissue or bone formation. In the presence of fibrous tissue, the fracture gap may be adequately stabilised to allow chondral tissue to form. With the increased stability, neovascularisation can occur, increasing tissue oxygen tension and allowing osteoblastic differentiation and bone formation [21]. The outcome of cementless fixation has clear similarities, with bone ingrowth occurring only in the presence of mechanical stability.

Factors Affecting Cementless Fixation

Successful osseo-integration of a cementless prosthesis occurs in three phases: stable initial fixation,

bone ingrowth and bone remodelling. Various factors may affect one or more of these phases and will be discussed.

Operative Technique

An essential requirement for successful cementless arthroplasty is immediate stability of the implant. Cameron et al. [22] studied the effect of motion on bone ingrowth into porous staples in rabbit tibiae. Micromotion was harmless but macromotion was not. Later Pilliar et al. [23] and Burke et al. [24] showed motion less than 150 μm was required to allow bone ingrowth. Stability of a prosthesis requires a tight fit. Implantation of an identically sized implant to the rasp or reamer used achieves line to line contact. In a cadaveric study [25], line to line insertion of an acetabular component resulted in micromotion of 150 μm compared with less motion when a press fit (1 mm under-reamed) insertion was employed. Furthermore, it is unlikely that an exact fit will be achieved with a line-to-line technique given the inconsistent nature of hand-held instruments, and experimental studies have shown fibrous tissue ingrowth with a gap of as little as 1 mm [26]. Finally, the strength of cancellous bone increases with increasing proximity to the endosteum. A prosthesis that fills the femoral canal in both the anteroposterior and mediolateral planes should therefore be selected (Fig 7.2).

Host Factors and Therapies

Great variations in the morphology of the proximal femur have been described [27, 28], resulting in a classification into types A, B or C (Fig 7.3).

Since stable initial fixation into the stovepipe (type C) femur is difficult to achieve, this anatomy is a relative contraindication to cementless femoral fixation.

In a comparison of patients with and without osteoporotic bone Dorr et al. [29] found no difference in clinical outcome at 5 years, although a difference in the bone remodelling response was seen which could affect the longer-term survival. A number of other bone diseases may interfere with initial stability, ingrowth or remodelling around a cementless prosthesis (Table 7.1).

The vascular compromise of avascular necrosis may impair ingrowth fixation either in the acute healing phase or later in the remodelling phase due to recurrent or progressive avascular episodes. This potential loss of fixation is applicable to both cemented and cementless designs.

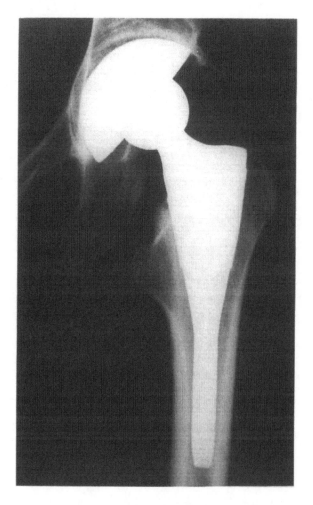

Fig. 7.2. A good canal fill ensures good bone support and improves the contact area between the ingrowth area on the prosthesis and the surrounding bone. The prosthesis has a slenderised stem (with a biodegradable centraliser) to reduce the flexural mismatch.

Bone loss is well known to occur with increasing age, and studies have shown profound differences both in the ability of bone to remodel with age and in the percentage of porous space ingrown by bone with increasing age [30]. The resultant decrease in

interfacial strength may extrapolate into higher failure rates with increasing age, although this may be offset by a commensurate reduction in the activity profile.

A number of therapies have been shown to inhibit bone formation including steroids, *cis*-platinum and agents employed to treat heterotopic ossification such as etidronate, indomethacin and gamma irradiation. Patients being treated with these agents would be less likely to osseo-integrate, and the consequent compromise of fixation would contribute to premature failure.

Prosthetic Factors

Materials

A biomaterial is defined as a non-viable material, used in a medical device, intended to interact with biological systems [32]. Biomaterials may be classified according to their chemistry into ceramics, metals, polymers and composites or according to the reaction induced in the host under optimum biomechanical conditions [33]. A connective tissue layer surrounds biotolerant implants; bioinert implants are characterised by direct contact between implant and bone and bioactive implants form a chemical bond with bone (Table 7.2).

The most commonly used metal implants in orthopaedic procedures are stainless steel, cobalt–chrome (Co–Cr), commercially pure (c.p.) titanium and titanium (Ti) alloy.

Stainless steel has been unsuccessful in cementless arthroplasty due to its poor corrosive properties [34]. Co–Cr alloys are the most fatigue resistant materials while Ti is superior with respect to corrosive resistance [35]. Ti has been shown to be particularly biocompatible [36] and has an elastic modulus nearer to that of bone than the other materials. Ti alloy has superior mechanical properties to c.p. Ti

Table 7.1. Effect of bone disease in initial stability and osseointegration

	Initial stability	Ossification
Osteoporosis	D	D
Osteomalacia	D	D
Paget's disease	D	D
Renal osteodystrophy	D	D
Avascular necrosis	D/N	D/N

D = deficient   N = normal

Table 7.2. Classification of biomaterials according to host response

Material	Class	Interface
Bone cement, stainless steel, Co–Cr alloy	Biotolerant	Connective tissue layer between implant and bone
Alumina, zirconia, carbon, titanium	Bioinert	Direct bone–implant contact
Hydroxyapatite, tricalcium phosphate, bioglasses	Bioactive	Chemical bonding

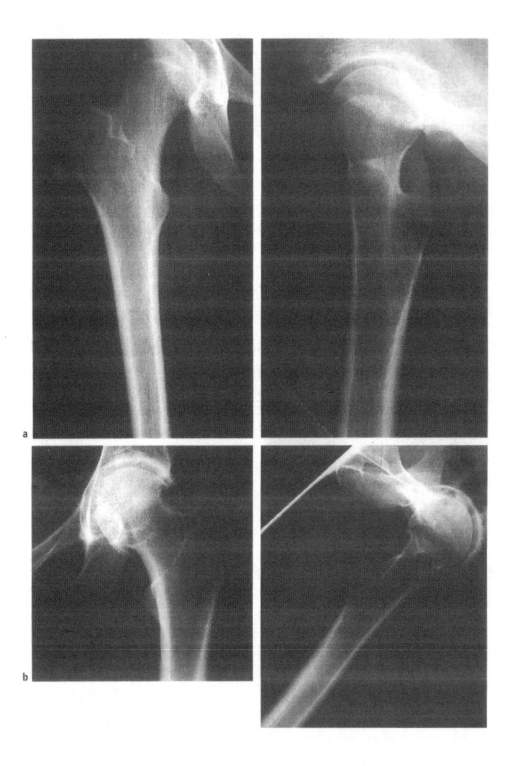

Fig. 7.3.   **a** Type A bone: "champagne flute" on AP and lateral radiograph. **b** Type B bone: "champagne flute" on AP only. "Stove pipe" appearance on lateral. **c** Type C bone: "stove pipe" appearance on both AP and lateral [27].

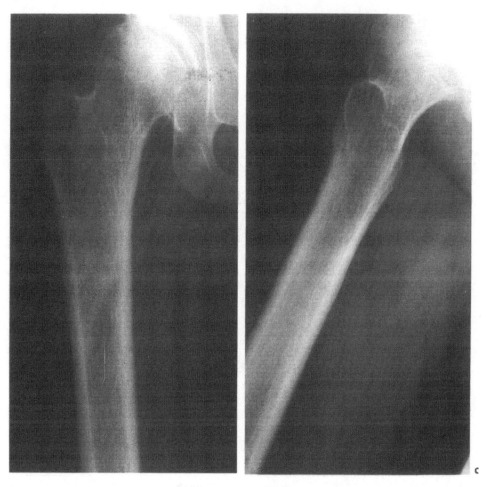

Fig. 7.3.   *(continued)*

with similar elastic modulus and corrosive resistance [37]. Ti is rapidly oxidised so that all Ti implants have a stable ceramic Ti oxide layer on their surface.

Surface Morphology

The mode of fixation of a cementless implant will be affected not only by the mechanical and material environment but also by the surface finish of the device. Smooth, irregular or fenestrated and porous surfaces have all been used. In all but the porous surface a layer of fibrous tissue between prosthesis and bone generally provides the fixation [38, 39]. In the presence of a biocompatible porous surface and a favourable mechanical environment, bone ingrowth will occur [40, 41]. A porous surface is one in which a series of interconnecting channels are formed by coating the metal substrate surface with a layer of small particles in the form of beads, fibre or powder (Fig. 7.4). Lower values of interfacial micromotion have been reported with porous surfaces compared

with smoother press fit surfaces [42]. This improves the likelihood of bone ingrowth but also achieves better stability if fibrous ingrowth occurs. For rapid ingrowth of bone and maximum fixation strength, a pore size in the range of 100 to 400 μm appears most effective [43]. These experiments were carried out in unloaded models and a slightly higher range may be more effective in a loaded application (Fig. 7.5). Further tests demonstrated superior fixation strength for implants with multiple particle layers [44]. In a multiple layered coating, however, there is an increased risk of debonding unless particle interconnectivity is maintained. If interconnectivity is too high the pore size decreases. The optimum volume fraction porosity to balance these factors is 30 to 40%.

Numerous metals, polymers and ceramic surfaces have been investigated and show similar ingrowth behaviour. Metallic coatings are the most commonly used types, applied by the sintering process, diffusion bonding or plasma spraying. Sintering is used to form a coating of beads of Co–Cr alloy or Ti alloy

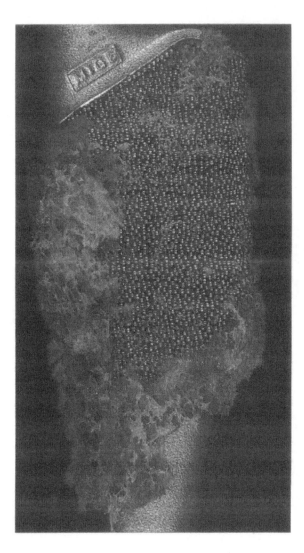

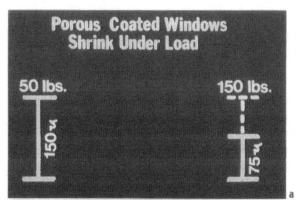

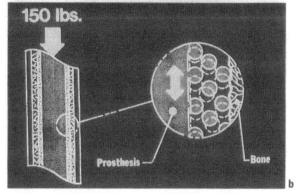

Fig. 7.5. Functional pore size: **a** the effect of loading; **b** the effect of differential movement between prosthesis and bone on actual pore size.

Fig. 7.4. A beaded, multilayered porous surface showing patchy bone ingrowth.

onto their respective material substrates. This process is carried out at high temperatures melting the beads onto the surface and may a cause a significant loss in fatigue strength of the substrate. This is particularly true of the Ti alloys. Diffusion bonding attaches Ti fibre onto a Ti alloy substrate and is performed under pressure at a lower temperature than sintering, avoiding the subsequent loss of strength. With the plasma spray technique a heated metal powder is sprayed onto the unheated substrate currently using powder and substrate of Ti alloy. The pore size obtained using the sintering technique ranges from 150–350 μm, while the fibre metal has a mean pore size of approximately 350 μm and the plasma spray approximately 300 μm. Loss of fixation of the coating to the substrate is rarely seen but

has been reported in bead coatings and is a sensitive test of implant stability. Metal ions are released from implant surfaces [45] and there are concerns over the increased surface area in porous implants although the significance is as yet unknown [46].

Lower modulus coatings on a narrow metal core are an attractive alternative since the decreased stiffness of the composite stem may result in less resorptive bone remodelling [47]. Clinical trials have however been disappointing due to debonding of the coating [48]. A new generation of fully coated low modulus composite stems are currently being evaluated (Fig 7.6).

The optimal extent of surface coating is unresolved. The original cementless components were fully coated resulting in bonding of the cortical diaphyseal bone to the coating – so called spot welding [15]. This distal fixation shields the proximal femur from loading resulting in proximal stress protection osteopenia. This proximal loss of bone density is felt by Engh et al. to be an indicator of a well-fixed stem and there is apparently no progression of bone loss after 2 years. Newer cementless designs have a reduced area of porous coating which is confined to

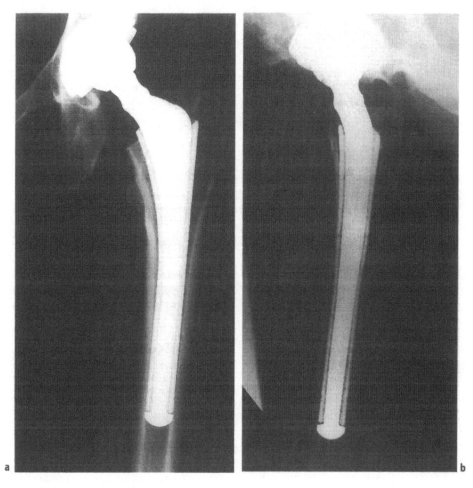

Fig. 7.6.a, b AP and lateral of a low modulus composite stem: the metal core is surrounded by a plastic polymer and the prosthesis is covered with a skin of titanium mesh.

the metaphyseal region of the implant. These therefore aim to achieve metaphyseal fixation of the implant, thereby avoiding stress shielding, while they also reduce the area for metal ion release and corrosion. Removal of proximally coated stems should also be easier if revision is required, although this is disputed. The cancellous hypertrophy seen with metaphyseal fixation has been termed the buttress support pattern and is first seen radiographically 1–2 years after surgery, progressing for a further 4 or 5 years. This is often associated with rounding off of the calcar. The incidence of thigh pain appears to vary with the degree of coating. Engh et al. [49] showed double the rate of thigh pain and radiographic loosening in proximally coated compared with fully coated designs. However extensive the coating, there is general agreement that the coating should be fully circumferential [50, 51]. Circumferential bone ingrowth restricts the access of particulate debris to the interface and thus prevents osteolysis.

Bioactive Surface Coatings

Human cadaveric retrievals of clinically well-performing implants have failed to show the expected bony ingrowth [52, 42]. This may be due to a number of factors including lack of direct contact between implant and bone [53] or excessive micromovement despite apparent stable initial fixation [24]. Attention has focused on the need for improved biological behaviour of implant materials to enhance bone ingrowth, with particular reference to calcium phosphate ceramics. HA has been most extensively studied as an implant coating. The development of plasma spraying of HA onto metal [54] overcame the problem of the low bending and shear strength of these ceramics. The quality of HA coatings is highly variable. The amount of HA lost is estimated at 15 μm in the first year after which stabilisation supposedly occurs if there is bone coverage [55, 56]. In a retrieval study by Bauer et al.

[57, 58] five HA-coated hip arthroplasties were analysed histologically. HA and bone were noted to be resorbed in areas where stresses were expected to be low but a uniform layer of HA and cancellous condensation were present in areas of stress transfer. A. Malcolm (1998, personal communication) has examined a cadaveric specimen 9 years after implantation, and reported complete resorption of the HA coating. However, he noted an intimate "custom-made" press fit with a completely stable implant.

A 50–75 µm coating is generally accepted as the optimum compromise to promote bone ongrowth and avoid rapid resorption while providing secure substrate fixation. It also avoids the obliteration of pores caused by a thicker coating on a porous surface [54]. Purity of the coating should be high (95–97%), crystallinity in the range 70–90% and calcium/phosphate ratio of 1:1.67. The bond strength between HA and substrate varies between 5 and 65 MPa depending on the substrate surface and HA quality, and failure between HA and substrate has been reported [59]. Application of HA onto a roughened or porous surface eliminates the peeling off seen with flat surfaces [60] demonstrating the importance of component design. Substrate fixation is enhanced by spraying on a precoat of titanium.

Histological studies of retrieved implants have demonstrated several stages in the osseo-integration of the implant. Osteoblasts differentiating from the loose connective tissue have invaded the bone marrow cavity a few weeks after implantation and synthesized an osteoid matrix on the coating, thus forming immature bone.

A series of studies by Soballe [61] comparing HA with Ti coating have shown the ability of HA coating on a porous surface to enhance the healing of gaps up to 2 mm, achieve stable fixation in porotic bone and eventual bony ingrowth in the presence of micromotion up to 500 µm. These observations were all improvements on the performance of the titanium coated implant.

Clinical studies of HA-coated prostheses are equally encouraging. Geesink [62] reported early results for 100 patients with an average age of 34 years. There were no loose stems and 92% were free of thigh pain with only one patient reporting activity-limiting pain. D'Antonio et al. [63] reviewed 436 hips with HA coatings. Activity-limiting pain was present in 1.4% of cases, there were two revisions (0.46%) for aseptic loosening and no further radiographically loose stems. Both series used roughened but not porous Ti alloy implants. Dorr et al. [64] reported an improvement in the buttress remodelling pattern when HA was sprayed onto a proximally porous coated stem and predict that these stems will be more durable in the long term.

Thus the advantages of HA coating include acceleration of osseo-integration, the enhanced ability of bone to bridge gaps of up to 2 mm, and the provision of a complete seal at the component bone interface. However concern remains about the possibility of resorption of HA, debonding from the substrate and a potential contribution to three body wear.

Summary

Cementless fixation aims to overcome the problem of long-term failure of cemented fixation, particularly in the younger, more active patient. The generally accepted goal is functional osseo-integration of the implant with proximal stress transfer to the femur. Component design variables and operative technique in addition to host factors will critically affect whether or not this goal is achieved. Long-term clinical studies are required to demonstrate the efficacy and durability of this mode of fixation.

References

1. Kerboull M. Cemented stems in young patients. In: Challenges in Total Hip Replacement. Smith and Nephew International Hip Conference, Lisbon, 1998; 22–24.
2. Chandler CN, Reineck FT, Wixson RL, McCarthy JC. Total hip replacement in patients younger than thirty years old. J Bone Joint Surg 1981;63B:1426–1429.
3. Cornell CN, Ranawat CS. Survivorship analysis of total hip replacements in a series of active patients who are less than fifty years old. J Bone Joint Surg 1986;68A:1430–1434.
4. Halley DK, Wroblewski BM. Long-term results of low-friction arthroplasty in patients 30 years of age or younger. Clin Orthop 1986;211:43–50.
5. Fornasier V, Wright J, Seligman J. The histomorphologic and morphometric study of asymptomatic hip arthroplasty. Clin Orthop 1991271:272–282.
6. Gates EI, Harris WH. Comparative fatigue behaviour of different bone cements. Clin Orthop 1984;189:294–299.
7. Halawa M, Lee A, Ling RSM. The shear strength of trabecular bone from the femur and some factors affecting the shear strength of the cement –bone interface. Arch Orthop Trauma Surg 1978;92:19–30.
8. Gruen TA, Amstutz HC. Effects of laminations and blood entrapment on the strength of acrylic bone cement. Clin Orthop 1976;119:250–255.
9. Linder L. Monomer leakage from polymerising acrylic bone cement. Clin Orthop 1976;119:242–249.
10. Mjoberg B, Petterson H, Rosenqvist R, Rydholm A. Bone cement, thermal injury and the radiolucent zone. Acta Orthop Scand 1984;55:597–600.
11. Jefferiss CD, Lee AJC, Ling RSM. Thermal aspects of self curing polymethylmethacrylate. J Bone Joint Surg 1975; 57B:511–518.
12. Cook SD, Walsh KA, Haddad RJ Jr. Interface mechanics and bone ingrowth into porous Co–Cr–Mo alloy implants. Clin Orthop 1985;193:271–280.
13. Maistrelli GL, Mahomed N, Garbuz D, Fornasier V, Harrington IJ, Binnington A. Hydroxyapatite coating on carbon composite hip implants in dogs. J Bone Joint Surg 1992;74B:452–456.

14. Walker PS, Onchi K, Kurosawa H, Rodger RF. Approaches to the interface problem in total joint arthroplasty. Clin Orthop 1984;182:99–108.

15. Engh CA, Bobyn VD, Glassman AJ. Porous-coated hip replacement. The factors governing bone-ingrowth, stress shielding and clinical results. J Bone Joint Surg 1987; 69B:45–55.

16. Maistrelli GL, Mahomed N, Fornasier V, Antonelli L, Li Y, Binnington A. Functional osseointegration of HA coated implants. J Arthroplasty 1993;8:549–554.

17. Schenk RK. Cytodynamics and histodynamics of primary bone repair. In: Lane JM (ed) Fracture healing. New York: Churchill Livingstone, 1987; 23–32.

18. Rahn BA, Gallinaro P, Baltensperger A, Perren SM. Primary bone healing. An experimental study in the rabbit. J Bone Joint Surg 1971;54:783–786.

19. Brown CC, McLaughlin RE, Balian G. Intramedullary bone repair and ingrowth into porous coated implants in the adult chicken: a histologic study and biochemical analysis of collagens. J Orthop Res 1989;7:316–325.

20. Perren SM. Physical and biological aspects of fracture healing with special reference to internal fixation. Clin Orthop 1979;138:175–196.

21. Bassett CAL, Hermann I. Influence of oxygen concentration and mechanical factors on differentiation of connective tissues in vitro. Nature 1961;190:460–461.

22. Cameron HU, Pilliar RM, MacNab I. The effect of movement on the bonding of porous metal to bone. J Biomed Mater Res 1973;7:301–311.

23. Pilliar RM, Lee JM, Maniatopoulos C. Observation on the effect of movement on bone ingrowth into porous surfaced implants. Clin Orthop 1986;208:108–113.

24. Burke DW, O'Connor DA, Zalenski EB, Jasty M, Harris WH. Micromotion of cemented and uncemented femoral components. J Bone Joint Surg 1991;73B:33–37.

25. Stiehl JB, MacMillan, Skrade DA. Mechanical stability of porous coated acetabular components in total hip arthroplasty. J Arthroplasty 1991;6:295–300.

26. Jasty M, O'Connor DO, Henshaw RM, Harrigan TP, Harris WH. Fit of the uncemented femoral component and the use of cement influence the strain transfer to the femoral cortex J Orthop Res 1994;12:648–656.

27. Dorr LD, Faugere MC, Mackel AM, Gruen TA, Bognar G, Malluche HH. Structural and cellular assessment of bone quality of proximal femur. Bone 1993;14:231–242.

28. Noble PC, Alexander JW, Lindahl LJ, Yew DT, Granberry WM, Tullos HS. The anatomic basis of femoral component design. Clin Orthop 1988;235:148–165.

29. Dorr LD, Arnala I, Faugere MC, Malluche HH. Five-year postoperative results of cemented femoral arthroplasty in patients with systemic bone disease. Clin Orthop 1990; 259:114–121.

30. Nakajima I, Dai KR, Kelly PJ, Chao PYS. The effect of age on bone ingrowth into titanium fiber metal segmental prosthesis: an experimental study in a canine model. Orthop Trans 1985;9:296–297.

31. Rivero DP, Skipor AK, Singh M, Urban RM, Galante JO. Effect of disodium etidronate (EHDP) on bone ingrowth in a porous material. Clin Orthop 1987;215:279–286.

32. Williams DF. Consensus and definitions in biomaterials. In: De Putter C, de Lange GL, De Groot K, Lee AJC (eds) Advances in biomaterials. Amsterdam: Elsevier, 1988; 8: 1–16.

33. Osborn JF, Newsley H. Dynamic aspects of the implant-bone interface. In: Heimke G (ed) Dental implants. Munich: Carl Hanser Verlag, 1980; 111–123.

34. Crowninshield R. An overview of prosthetic materials for fixation. Clin Orthop 1988;235:166–172.

35. Cohen J, Wulff J. Clinical failure caused by corrosion of a

vitallium plate. J Bone Joint Surg 1972;54B:617–628.

36. Albrektsson T, Branemark P-I, Hansson HA, Lindstrom J. Osseointegrated titanium implants: requirements for ensuring a long-lasting, direct bone anchorage in man. Acta Orthop Scand 1981;52:155–170.

37. Keller JC, Lautenschlager EP. Metals and alloys. In: Von Recum AF (ed) Handbook of biomaterials evaluation. Scientific, technical and clinical testing of implant materials. New York: Macmillan, 1986; 3–23.

38. Morscher EW. Cementless total hip arthroplasty. Clin Orthop 1983;181:76–91.

39. Ring PA. Ring UPM total hip arthroplasty. Clin Orthop 1983;176:115–123.

40. Spector M. Bone ingrowth into porous metals. In: Williams DF (ed) Biocompatibility of orthopaedic implants. Boca Raton FL: CRC Press, 1982; I:89.

41. Spector M. Bone ingrowth into porous polymers. In: Williams DF (ed) Biocompatibility of orthopaedic implants. Boca Raton FL: CRC Press, 1982; II:55.

42. Cook SD, Thomas KA, Haddad RJ Jr. Histologic analysis of retrieved human porous coated total joint components. Clin Orthop 1988;234:90–101.

43. Bobyn JD, Pilliar RM, Cameron HU, Weatherly GC. The optimum pore size for the fixation of porous surfaced metal implants. Clin Orthop 1980;150:263–270.

44. Bobyn JD, Pilliar RM, Cameron HU, Weatherly GC, Kent GM. The effect of porous surface configuration on the tensile strength of fixation of implants. Clin Orthop 1980;149: 291–298.

45. Agins HJ, Alcock NW, Bensal M et al. Metallic wear in failed titanium – alloy total hip replacement. J Bone Joint Surg 1988;70B 1:347–356.

46. Jacobs JJ, Skipor AK, Black J, Urban RM, Galante JO. Release and examination of metal in patients who have a total hip replacement component made of titanium base alloy. J Bone Joint Surg 1991;73A:1475–1486.

47. Maistrelli GL. Polymers in orthopaedics. In: Cameron HU (ed) Bone implant interface. St. Louis MO: Mosby,1994; 169–179.

48. Tullos HS, McCaskill BL, Dickey R, Davidson J. Total hip arthroplasty with a low-modulus porous coated femoral component. J Bone Joint Surg 1984;66A 1:888–898.

49. Engh CA, O'Connor D, Jasty M, McGovern TF, Bobyn JD, Harris WH. Quantification of implant micromotion, strain shielding and bone resorption with porous coated prosthesis. Clin Orthop 1992;285:13–29.

50. Hubble MJ, Eldridge JD, Smith EJ, Learmonth ID, Harris YM. Patterns of osteolysis in two different cementless total hip arthroplasties. Hip Int 1997;7:65–69.

51. Schmalzried TP, Jasty M, Harris WH. Periprosthetic bone loss in THA. Polyethylene wear debris and the concept of the effective joint space. J Bone Joint Surg 1992;74A:849–861.

52. Bobyn JD, Engh CA. Human histology of the bone–porous metal implant interface. Orthopaedics 1984;7:1410–1421.

53. Schimmel J-W, Huiskes R. Primary fit of the Lord cementless total hip. A geometric study in cadavers. Acta Orthop Scand 1988;59:638–642.

54. De Groot K, Geesink RGT, Klein CPAT, Serekian P. Plasma sprayed coatings of hydroxyapatite. J Biomed Mater Res 1987;21:1375–138.

55. Van Blitterswiik CA, Grote JJ, Kuypers W, Daems WT, de Groot K. Macropore tissue ingrowth: a quantitative study on hydroxyapatite ceramic. Biomaterials 1986;7:137–143.

56. Geesink RGT, De Groot K, Klein CPAT. Bone bonding to apatite coated stems. J Bone Joint Surg 1988;70B:17–22.

57. Bauer TW, Geesink RC, Zimmerman R, McMahon JT. Hydroxyapatite coated femoral stems. Histological analysis of components retrieved at autopsy. J Bone Joint Surg 1991;73A:1439–1452.

58. Bauer TW, Stulberg BN, Ming J, Geesink RG. Uncemented acetabular components: histologic analysis of retrieved hydroxyapatite coated and porous implants. J Arthroplasty 1993;8:167–177.

59. Thomas KA, Kay JF, Cook SD, Jarcho M. The effect of surface macrotexture and hydroxyapatite coating on the mechanical strengths and histological profiles of titanium implant materials. J Biomed Mater Res 1987;21:1395–1414.

60. Oonishi H, Tsuji E, Ishimaru H, Yamamoto M, Delecrin J. Comparative effects of HAp coated on flat and porous metal surfaces. In: Heimke G (ed) Bioceramics. Cologne: German Ceramic Society, 1990; 286–293.

61. Soballe K. Hydroxyapatite ceramic coating for bone implant fixation. Mechanical and histological studies in dogs. Acta Orthop Scand Suppl 1993;255:1–58.

62. Geesink RG. Hydroxyapatite-coated total hip prosthesis. Two year clinical and roentgenographic results of 100 cases. Clin Orthop 1990;261:39–58.

63. D'Antonio JA, Capello WN, Jaffe WL. Hydroxyapatite-coated hip implants. Multicenter three-year clinical and roentgenographic results. Clin Orthop 1992;285:102–115.

64. Dorr LD, Wan Z, Seng M, Ranawat A. Bilateral total hip arthroplasty comparing hydroxyapatite coating to porous-coated fixation. J Arthroplasty 1998;13:729–736.

8. Importance of Prosthesis Design and Surface Structure for the Primary and Secondary Stability of Uncemented Hip Joint Prostheses

S. Weller, A. Braun, J.C. Gellrich and U. Gross

Introduction

Primary stability and survival, i.e. long-term fixation, of a hip joint prosthesis is determined by the implant material, the bone stock serving as the implant bed, and the interaction between the implant material and the bone stock. The fate of a cementless artificial joint is decided at the interface or boundary between the bone and the implant, where living tissue meets bioinert (i.e. non-living) material. Numerous causes of loosening of aseptic implants have been identified. Invariably, they involve one of the following three major complexes acting at the interface (Fig. 8.1a, b):

1. implant material, implant design and surface structure;
2. bone stock, bone quality and form fit of the implant;
3. interactions between the bone stock – i.e. the implant bed – and the implant.

The implant must be strong enough to withstand changing load peaks and long-term loading. It must be biocompatible, i.e. tolerated by the tissue. The contact area between the implant and the bone must be as large as possible and the fit as tight as possible.

Bone, the living material serving as the biological substrate for the implant, is continuously remodelled as a result of the constantly changing loads imposed by the implant. The quality and load-bearing capability of bone vary greatly, being adversely affected by advancing age and beneficially affected by physical activity

The factors which may have a detrimental effect on this biological remodelling over the long term are: reactions of the bone stock to material particles abraded from the implant, toxic or thermal damage and inadequate primary stability. The latter may have its origin in the surgical technique or implant design and material.

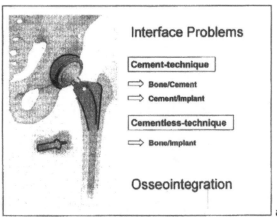

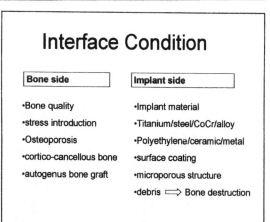

Fig. 8.1.a, b Interface problems and interface conditions.

Cemented or Uncemented Stabilisation

Charnley revolutionised total hip replacement in the late 1950s with the introduction of the "low friction principle" and cemented fixation of prosthetic components. This had a tremendous effect on the field of coxarthroplasty and promoted the widespread use of hip joint implants.

There have been numerous reports of the impressive long-term results [11, 16, 18, 19, 31, 36, 37, 39, 42, 44, 45, 46–48, 55, 68, 69] achieved with cemented prostheses. However there has been a commensurate increase in the number of cases of aseptic loosening associated with cemented fixation of prosthetic components. On occasions this loosening and osteolysis presents a challenging technical problem, and extensive loss of bone stock may be associated with a compromised circulation in the acetabular region (Fig. 8.2a, b, c).

The use of bone cement, in the hands of surgeons skilled in handling this material, indisputably guarantees the good form fit required at the interface as well as providing optimal primary stability. This is a definite advantage, especially in older patients with poor bone quality (e.g. patients suffering from osteoporosis caused by inactivity, mineralisation disorders, chronic inflammation, etc.) and in patients with delayed or impaired bone remodelling. On the other hand, bone cement exhibits limited stability and durability (vibration resistance) – especially with respect to long-term fixation – as a result of the so-called ageing processes. The bone stock may also be compromised by thermal damage resulting in impaired circulation, the toxic effects of free monomers, and infection [2, 6, 16, 33, 41] (Fig. 8.3a, b).

These negative experiences – together with the steadily increasing number of prostheses being implanted in young patients with a longer life expectancy and a higher activity profile – prompted the development of uncemented implant techniques and ushered in the "second era of joint prostheses". This does not mean, however, that bone cement has been discarded. As general life expectancy rises – and with it the average age of implant recipients – the percentage of patients with poor bone stock, in particular patients with post-traumatic pathology (e.g. femoral neck fractures), has increased dramatically [17, 18, 34, 41, 47, 50, 61]. There is thus still considerable scope for cemented implantation.

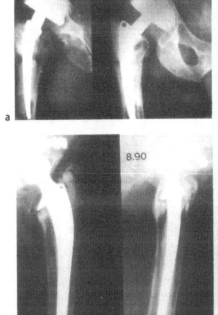

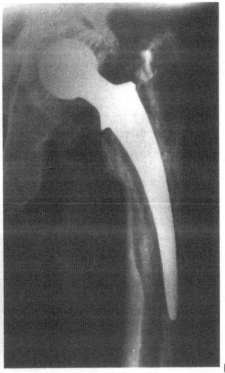

Fig. 8.2a, b, c Aseptic loosening after cemented implantation. Extensive bone defects with impaired circulation.

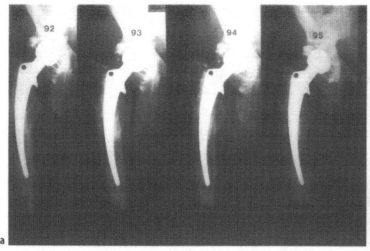
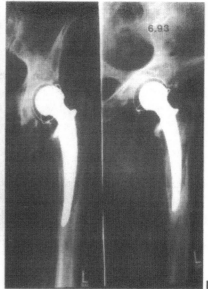

Fig. 8.3.a, b   Ageing process of bone cement with "cystic granuloma".

General Criteria for Hip Joint Implants

As long as the main problem influencing durable prosthetic fixation, namely the difficulty of creating a long-lasting bond between living tissue and bio-inert material, remains fundamentally unresolved, a decision will have to be made in each individual case whether to employ uncemented or cemented implant techniques [47, 49, 53, 59]. The principal factors influencing this decision are the patient's age and life expectancy as well as the load-bearing capability and overall quality of his or her bones.

On the basis of past experience, the following general clinical criteria have been established for hip joint implant systems [5, 61, 62]:

- A good implant system must exhibit universal applicability, i.e. it must be suitable for cemented, uncemented and revision implants, etc.
- The prosthesis design, including material composition and surface structure, must be optimal.
- The system must include a simple and easily surveyable range of instruments containing all tools needed to perform the various implantation procedures.
- The surgical procedures must be based on "biological implantation techniques" ensuring maximum conservation of bone and tissue.
- The implants must exhibit high primary and secondary stability, even for rotation.
- The cost/benefit ratio must be appropriate (long-term implants!).

It is still very difficult to test and evaluate the quality of a prosthesis, the surgical approach and fixation technique used for its implantation, and predict the anticipated survival rate. This is because the clinical symptoms of aseptic loosening are generally not apparent until after approximately 5–7 years. We now accept that it is not possible to make comprehensive statements about the quality of a prosthesis system until about 10 years after implantation, at the earliest, on the basis of data obtained from patients who have taken part in all the follow-up examinations. This is why the advantages of design changes to uncemented implants which alter the stability in bone, must yet again be shown to be beneficial and efficacious [35, 36, 59, 61].

Special Features of the BiCONTACT Hip Joint Implant System

The BiCONTACT hip joint implant system (Fig. 8.4a, b) is a modular system containing prostheses in graduated sizes and offering options for cemented and uncemented fixation of prosthetic components; it also includes alternatives for patients with hip joint dysplasia and patients requiring revision surgery. It thus satisfies the criterion of universal applicability. The external form or design of the implant components in the contact area (interface) is the same for all variants. In prostheses intended for uncemented fixation, the surface of the contact zone has been

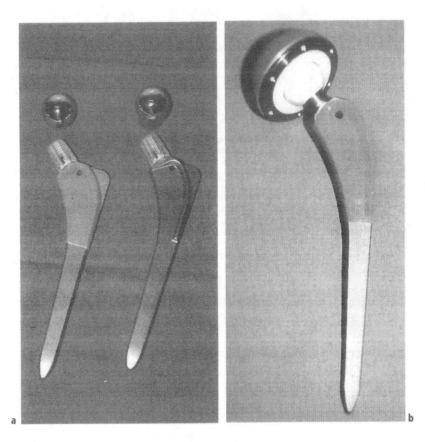

Fig. 8.4.a, b   BiCONTACT hip endoprosthesis system with special features for a cemented as well as uncemented implantation technique.

enlarged by a microporous pure titanium coating (Plasmapore) in order to promote bone ongrowth and ingrowth, i.e. the osseo-integration of the prosthesis [7, 15, 20, 24, 50, 62, 63]. The surgeon thus has the possibility, up to the definitive implantation of the implant, of modifying the fixation technique to suit the conditions encountered at the surgical site. Such a "switchover" may become necessary unexpectedly, for example, as a result of an acute toxic cardiovascular reaction caused by fixation of the acetabular cup with bone cement. A surgeon faced with this kind of critical situation will surely decide to continue the operation with uncemented implantation of stem components to be on the safe side. In other cases, where poor quality bone is unexpectedly encountered (e.g. patients with osteoporosis), a quick decision may be made to switch to cemented fixation because of the higher primary stability it offers [19].

During the R&D work on the BiCONTACT prosthesis, special emphasis was placed on developing a "biological" implantation technique which would, in accordance with the basic requirements listed above, preserve bone and tissue as far as possible. This

consideration applies equally to all the implantation techniques. This system was developed as a result of the experience gained in recent years during numerous revisions of prostheses, which were accompanied in many cases by substantial bone defects (Fig. 8.5a, b). It should always be remembered that during every primary implantation procedure and at every revision operation, the surgeon must consider the possibility and implications of the next prosthesis replacement.

Design Considerations (BiCONTACT Endoprosthesis System)

A modular osteoprofiler system is employed to conserve healthy bone and to compact cancellous bone in the femoral and acetabular regions of the hip joint (Fig. 8.6a–h). This ensures an optimal form fit of the implant, which encourages bone ingrowth and ongrowth; it also guarantees an optimal transfer

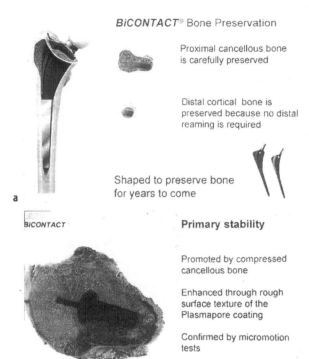

BiCONTACT® Bone Preservation

Proximal cancellous bone
is carefully preserved

Distal cortical bone is
preserved because no distal
reaming is required

Shaped to preserve bone
for years to come

Primary stability

Promoted by compressed
cancellous bone

Enhanced through rough
surface texture of the
Plasmapore coating

Confirmed by micromotion
tests

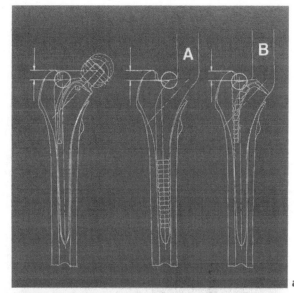

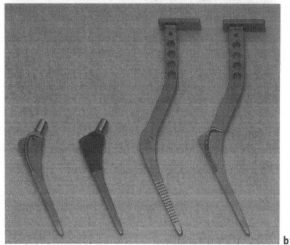

of forces. A distal tooth A-osteoprofiler is used to shape the medullary cavity; a series of these tools is inserted with sequentially increasing size. The lateral edge of the osteoprofiler compacts and compresses the intertrochanteric cancellous bone. A similar technique is used when the acetabular cup (plasma cup with a press fit) or a screw ring are inserted [50, 61, 62] (Fig. 8.6a, b).

The B-osteoprofiler is subsequently hammered into the compacted bone structure in the proximal femur with light blows. It precisely cuts the bony bed to accommodate the design features which will support the prosthesis stem. This stem has a special design: the dorsal anti-rotation fin and the lateral fixation fins improve rotational stability in addition to enlarging the prosthesis surface. After the prosthesis stem has been inserted, additional bone chips taken from the resected femoral head are placed in the resected area in order to achieve a tight bone contact [55, 61] (Fig. 8.7a–f, Fig. 8.5b).

Load transfer with "press fit" stability takes place exclusively in the intertrochanteric region in the proximal femur. A distal press fit of the prosthesis stem is not sought. This would lead to proximal stress protection which could ultimately cause troublesome

thigh pain and implant loosening. In addition, micromovements in the distal third of the prosthesis stem ensure a tight fit of the proximal region of the body of the prosthesis where the load is transferred to bone. This biomechanical constellation is demonstrated in selected cases from the patient group participating in the clinical follow-up; it is characterised by a small lucency, with a local sclerotic reaction occurring in the bone at the tip of the prosthetic stem with an otherwise asymptomatic stable implant which demonstrates the radiographic features of secure fixation (Fig. 8.8a, b).

The finely graduated implant sizes, the slightly conical stem form, the wide medial boundary surfaces and the elements for rotational stability (e.g.

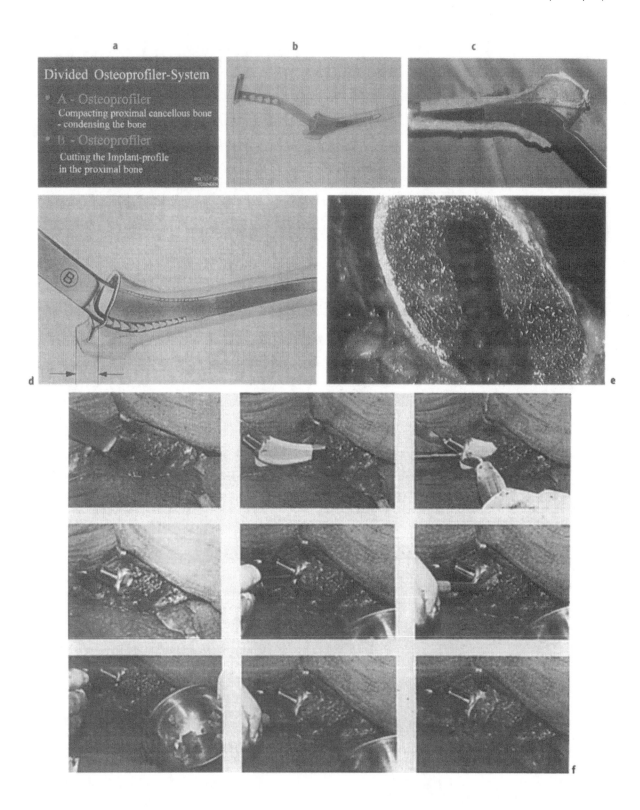

Fig 8.7.a–f   Divided osteoprofilers (A+B) to achieve close contacts of the components in the interface.

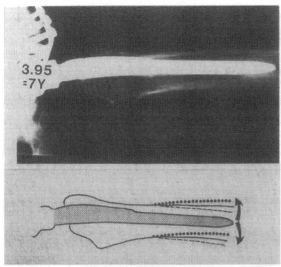

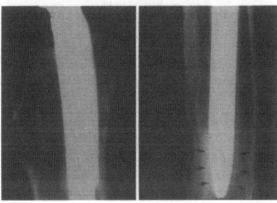

Fig. 8.8.a, b Proximal stress introduction with no loosening signs after 7 years. Distal micromotion between rigid implant and elastic bone. Local bone sclerosis.

lateral supporting surface, antirotation fin) guarantee a large area of support in the cancellous and cortical implant bed. The enlargement of the implant surface by a porous coating, with distribution of pressure forces at the implant-bone interface, encourages osseo-integration of the prosthesis. In this context, the microporous pure titanium coating (Plasmapore) has proved to be an effective and efficient catalyst of the bone ongrowth required for durable osseointegration.

Numerous studies have been conducted to find an optimal surface coating for cementless prosthetic components (stem and acetabular cup). The excellent ongrowth and ingrowth of bone achieved by the pure titanium Plasmapore coating has been demonstrated repeatedly in vitro and confirmed by clinical observations. However, the extent to which bone ongrowth and firm fixation can be further enhanced by various coating combinations, in

particular the addition of hydroxyapatite to a microporous metallic coating, still needs to be further explored [20, 50, 61].

Interaction Between Bone Mass and Implant

The fact that bone reacts to changes in its functional stress also applies with endoprosthesis implantation. In accordance with Wolff's law [67], a reduction in bone stress results in a reduction in bone mass and an increase in bone stress to an increase in bone mass. This adaptation of bone to the physical demands placed upon it is known as "bone remodelling" and may manifest itself in a modification in its density – "internal remodelling" – (Fig. 8.9a–d) and its circumference (Fig. 8.10a, b) [20, 25, 40, 54]. An essential feature of bony integration in cementless stems was proposed by Engh et al. in 1990 [21]. They identified this as the presence of new bone formation or "spot welds" which bridge the endosteal surface of the bone and the stem in the area of the proximal coating.

The BiCONTACT prosthesis stem (Fig. 8.4a, b) is designed for proximal fixation in the femur during cement-free implantation. The high primary and secondary stability achieved provides a firmer prosthesis–bone contact in the coated portion of the prosthesis stem, so that the load is transmitted from the prosthesis to the proximal femur (and similarly from the acetabular component to the pelvic bone). The plasma-coated portion of the prosthetic components provokes cancellous ingrowth and anchoring of the implant, thus providing secondary stability of the implant.

Animal Experiments

The basic work on the interaction of metallic surface structuring of cement-free endoprosthetic implants and bone tissue was published by Cameron et al. in 1973 [10] and Bobyn et al. in 1980 [8]. On the basis of this research, nearly all cement-free endoprostheses are now provided with a suitable surface for bone apposition (ongrowth).

It is important to distinguish fundamentally between roughened and fine textured surface structures when considering metallic surfaces. Titanium with a surface roughness of $R_t \sim 40$–50 μm is principally used as a roughened surface in clinical practice. A wide range of technical variations of the fine textured surfaces exist with pore sizes of 20 to 500 μm and with different porosities which, in the

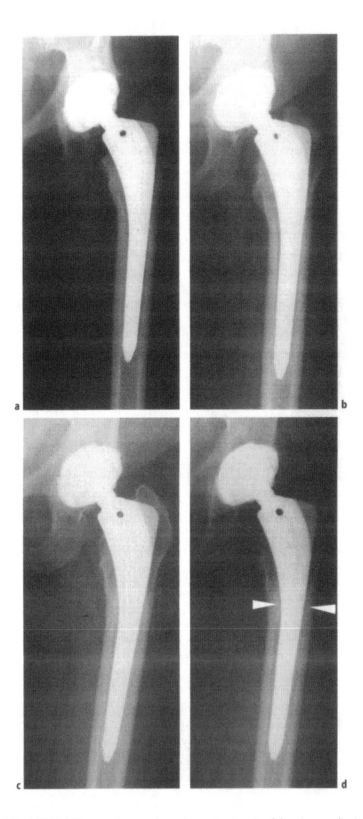

Fig. 8.9. "Internal remodelling". BiCONTACT-stem – 5 year progress observation. Atrophy of the calcar, condensing of bone mass (arrow) in the distal area of the Plasmapore coating as the expression of a maximum load transmission in this area. **a** postoperative, **b** 3 months postoperatively, **c** 3 years postoperatively, **d** 5 years postoperatively.

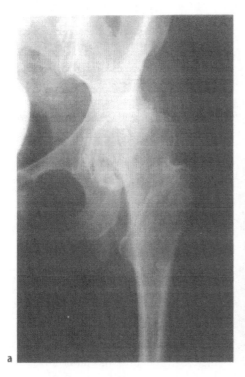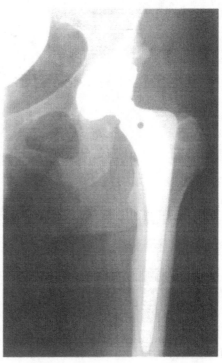

Fig. 8.10. "External remodelling". Dysplasia-arthrosis of the hip. BiCONTACT – progress observation over 5 years. High distal load transmission with a narrow femoral bone marrow cavity results in reactive increase in the peripheral cortical bone mass. **a** Preoperative; **b** 5 years post-operatively.

case of titanium and cobalt–chrome materials, have evolved over many years of clinical experience.

The results of cement-free hip joint prostheses obtained by Bülow et al. [9] (roughened titanium surface), Engh et al. [23] (CoCr-circumferential coating), and Mallory et al. [43] (titanium plasma spray) document survival rates of 96 to 98% with good radiological appearances of the stem components at subsequent follow-up of between 6 and 11 years. Identical experience with the BiCONTACT stem and the Plasmapore coating described in this report was presented in the context of a multicentre study by Asmuth et al. in 1998 [4].

Evidently, a judicious combination of the different types of surface combined with an appropriate biomechanical anchoring system was present in all the above hip joint prostheses.

Coating with microporous titanium provides a fine textured metallic surface which is employed by various manufacturers for the surface texturing of articular endoprostheses. The Plasmapore coating developed in the 1980s (vacuum manufacturing process) revealed pore sizes of 50–200 μm [24, 65]. The overall microporosity of 37.3% is composed of 13.7% with a pore size less than 50 μm, 9.6% between 50 and 100 μm and 14% between 100 and 200 μm (Fig. 8.11a, b).

The suitability of Plasmapore coating with the defined parameters for pore size and porosity was investigated by Gross in 1985 [30] in comparative animal experiments in the femoral condyles of Chinchilla rabbits and published by Winkler-Gniewek in 1989 [66]. Test cylinders with a smooth surface ($R_t = 1$ μm), a roughened surface ($R_t = 20$ μm) and a Plasmapore surface ($R_t = 100$ μm) were tested with an implantation time of 12 and 24 weeks. In addition to the histological analysis of the preparations (Fig. 8.12a–c), biomechanical substraction tests were performed (Fig. 8.13, Table 8.1). Distinctly different anchoring of the implants was demonstrated. In the biomechanical test in the interface between cancellous bone and the implant surface only the plasma-coated specimens showed subtraction values that were not zero (Table 8.1). In these biomechanical tests, the interface anchoring forces acting vertically to the implant surface were measured, in contrast to the pull-out tests (measurement of shear force) usually performed until then.

Whilst porosity and pore size affect the capacity for ongrowth and ingrowth of bone, the extreme roughness of the Plasmapore coating is also an important parameter influencing the primary stable anchoring of the implant. Comparative studies of cementless

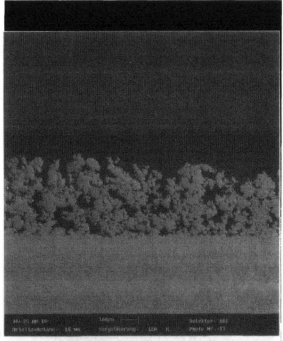

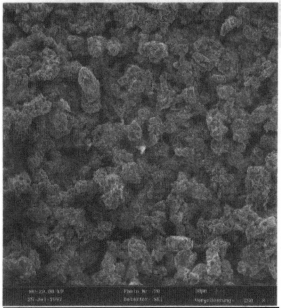

Fig. 8.11. **a** Plasmapore coating in cross-section. **b** View of Plasmapore coating.

Table 8.1. Results of tensile strength tests in animal experiments

Test sample	Surface roughness R1 (μm)	Number of samples N	Position time (days)	Mean tensile strength ± SD (N/mm²)	
Titanium	1	10	84	0	
Titanium	20	10	84	0	
Titanium	20	10	168	0	
Titanium plasmapore	100	10	84	5.53 ±	0.4
Titanium plasmapore	100	10	168	3.32 ±	0.82
Titanium plasmapore	100	71	168	4.47 ±	0.55

ened surfaces [27]. This supports the reported benefits of the use of a combination of hydroxyapatite with finely textured metallic surfaces (combination coatings). These developments flowed from the less favourable substrate interface conditions reported for ceramic coatings against a roughened prosthesis than with metallic surface coatings. Comparative histological and biomechanical trials by David et al. [14, 15] analysed the mechanical and histological interface conditions with different types of coating in animal experiments.

With the combination of a microtextured metallic surface and a thin coat of hydroxyapatite, the bioactive characteristics of the hydroxyapatite would enhance osseo-integration at the surface during the primary bone contact phase. Subsequently the good mechanical characteristics of microporous coatings would provide secondary stability. The place of combination coatings is currently still being evaluated and has still to demonstrate the desired advantages at the bone-implant interface (Fig. 8.14).

Histological Tests on Plasmapore Explants

press-fit sockets [51] confirm these important characteristics of the microporously textured surfaces. The process of plasma coating of implants implies fundamentally fewer restrictions on implant design than with other surface textures. It should be noted that reported interface stresses refer to osseo-integrated surfaces and not to loose implants.

Very good midterm clinical results have been reported with the use of hydroxyapatite on rough-

It was possible to document the intimate bond between bone and the microporous Plasmapore surface and demonstrate "bony ingrowth or ongrowth" on microscopic examination of individual joint endoprosthetic explants (Fig. 8.15). It was also possible to confirm these results on histological analysis of a BiCONTACT stem 9 months after implantation (Fig. 8.16). Reviewing a stem implanted on the left side, there was a macroscopically noticeable difference between the different bone apposition on the anterior surface of the prosthesis (less bone apposition) compared with the posterior surface (marked bone apposition). This

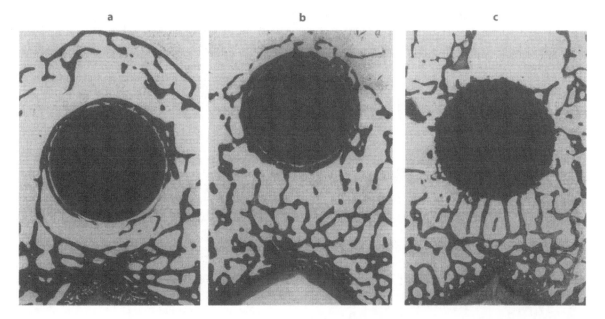

Fig. 8.12. Specimen implant anchoring preparations in animal experiments. **a** Flat titanium cylinder ($R_t = 1$ μm); **b** rough titanium cylinder ($R_t = 20$ μm) **c** Plasmapore titanium cylinder ($R_t = 100$ μm).

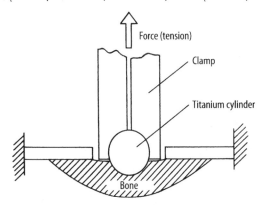

Fig. 8.13. Schematic drawing of biomechanical testing of implant anchoring.

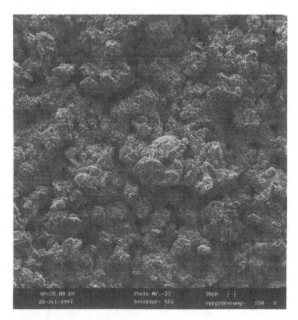

Fig. 8.14. Plasmapore with hydroxylapatite combination coating.

explant was also histologically analysed. It was possible to demonstrate how impressive bone ongrowth occurs around the prosthesis as early as 9 months after implantation (Fig. 8.17a,b). The following constituents were identified: Plasmapore coating = 1, lamellar bone trabeculae = 2, osteoid matrix = 3 and fatty bone marrow = 4.

Further knowledge of the bony integration of a Plasmapore coated BiCONTACT stem was obtained from a preparation in which it was possible to process the complete prosthesis/bone composite. This involved an amputation specimen following partial hemipelvectomy for local soft tissue recurrence of a primary clear cell chondrosarcoma of the femoral head 3 months after implantation of a cementless BiCONTACT stem (Fig. 8.18). The implant was left in bone, embedded in the non-decalcified state in synthetic material and sectioned with a saw microtome (Fig. 8.19).

The histological analyses (Fig. 8.20) of the interface confirm that, in accordance with the BiCONTACT design, direct contact between the Plasmapore-coated stem and cancellous bone occurs in the medial proximal area and supportively in the region of the lateral and anti-rotation wings (Fig. 8.21). The tissue around the implant demonstrates good viability with active new bone formation. In the medial proximal area, the contact between implant and bone amounts

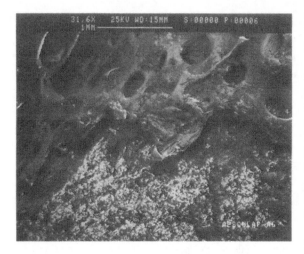

Fig. 8.15. Scanning electron microscope recording of an explant with bone–Plasmapore contact.

to approximately one fifth of the medial prosthesis surface (some 120 mm^2). The bone grows onto and into the Plasmapore coating in this contact area (Fig. 8.22). The thickness of the trabeculae is approximately 0.3 mm. Direct bone contact exists only in the distal portion of the coating on the anterior and posterior surfaces of the prosthesis (Fig. 8.21). Despite a good blood supply an inflammatory reaction was not observed.

Less bone contact is present on the lateral wing and the trabeculae are arranged vertically to the surface of the prosthesis. Isolated bone contact occurs on the posterolateral wings (Fig. 8.23). A very strong medial bone structure was noted in the distal Plasmapore-coated area with gradual transition from trabecular to cortical bone (Fig. 8.21). No implant bone contact is present in the distal uncoated prosthesis stem (Fig. 8.24). The load is therefore transmitted to the bone mainly through the medial interface of the prosthesis.

Histological examination three months after implantation of a BiCONTACT stem shows stable bony integration of the prosthesis. The number and thickness of the bone trabeculae ingrown in the Plasmapore coating on the medial surface of the

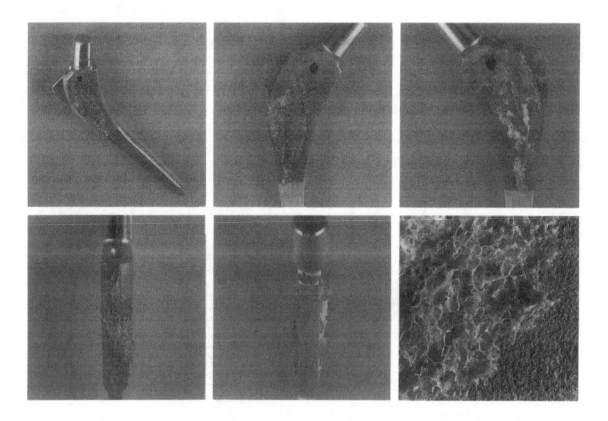

Fig. 8.16. BiCONTACT shaft explant 9 months postoperatively with varying bone contact.

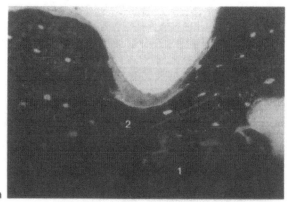

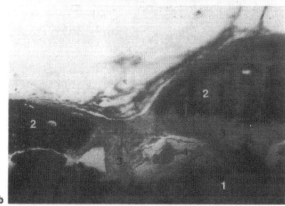

Fig. 8.17. Histological details on bone contact of the Plasmapore surface 9 months postoperatively. **a** Bony anchoring in the pores of the Plasmapore coating; 1 = Plasmapore coating, 2 = bone trabecula. **b** Foot-shaped formation of membranous bone between the trabecular structure of the osteoid matrix; 1 = Plasmapore coating, 2 = bone trabecula, 3 = osteoid matrix, 4 = fatty bone marrow.

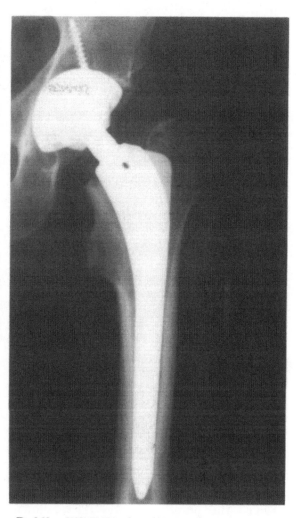

Fig. 8.18. BiCONTACT implant of hip 3 months postoperatively.

prosthesis as shown on histological examination represents a direct adaptation of the peri-prosthetic bone to the regional loads applied. This is in accordance with Wolff's law[67]. If one takes the prosthesis design, the anatomy of the proximal femur and the results of the histological examination three months after surgery into account, any sinkage of a BiCONTACT stem must be accepted as loosening. The histological results indicate that the greatest bony integration of the prosthesis is to be found in the distal half of the Plasmapore coating (see also Fig. 8.9d). This fact is supported by X-ray observation of the course of bone integration reported by Engh et al. in 1994 [22] and Gellrich in 1998 [28, 29]. The lack of bony integration of the smooth distal part of the stem allows micromovement. The histological results do not contradict our osteodensitometric results, which show an approximately 19% reduction in periprosthetic bone density in Gruen zones 1 and 7 in the first 6 months. It is conceivable

that bone trabeculae not subjected to stress undergo atrophy in the early post-operative period.

Periprosthetic Bone Reaction to Cementless Implantation of the BiCONTACT Stem

Imaging of the periprosthetic bone provides information regarding bone turnover and the interaction between the implant and the surrounding bone mass. Although conventional radiography can only detect a change in bone-mineral density in excess of 30%, it has proved useful in monitoring bone remodelling. The extent of the resorptive and appositional bone remodelling (Figs 8.9 and 8.10) depends on a variety of factors, including prosthesis design, surface coating and prosthesis size.

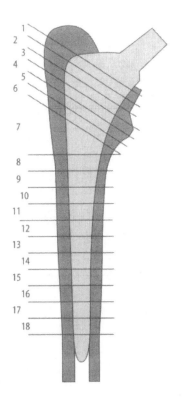

Fig. 8.19. Cut levels with the saw microtome.

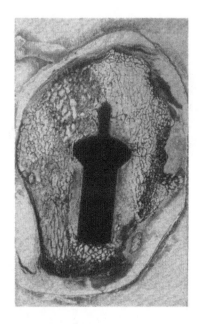

Fig. 8.20. Histological tests on the proximal interface of the BiCONTACT stem. Medial and lateral direct implant-bone contact (cut level 3).

The radiological sign suggestive of osseo-integration of cement-free stem prostheses is the endosteal presence of bone condensations – so-called "spot welds" – in the area of porous coating of the stem. This usually occurs at the transition between coated and uncoated prosthetic surfaces. This area is found in stems with metaphyseal coating and proximal load transfer at the isthmus of the femur, where the endosteal surface of the cortex and the implant are juxtaposed (Fig. 8.9d). This radiological sign is not, however, detectable in all cases with successful bony integration. In 50 BiCONTACT stems, the radiologically visible endosteal zone of bone condensation in the area of the transition from Plasmapore-coated to uncoated prosthesis surface was observed in only 30.6% of cases at 1 year after implantation.

It is difficult to interpret condensation of new bone growth around the tip of cementless prostheses. Cementless stems which rely on proximal anchoring are associated with relative movement of the distal uncoated part of the stem which produces these bone reactions. Loosening of the implant should only be suspected with progressive bone component lucency and with stem sinkage. The

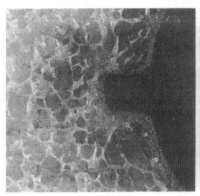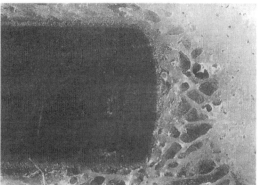

Fig. 8.21. Optimum bony integration in the middle and distal portion of the Plasmapore coating (cut level 5).

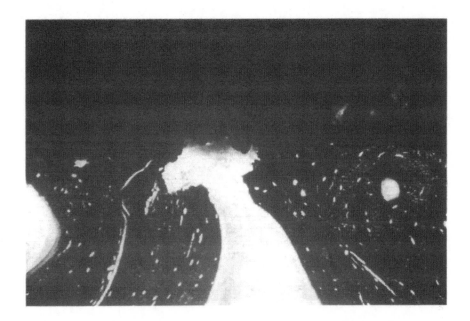

Fig. 8.22.   The bone grows in the contact zones and in the Plasmapore coating (cut level 3).

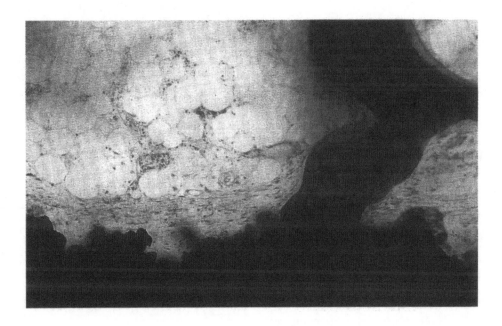

Fig. 8.23.   Isolated bone contact with the prosthesis on the posterolateral wing (cut level 3).

absence of lysis in the area of the porous coating of a cement-free stem is considered, together with the so-called "spot welds", as an indication of osseointegration of the implant [21]. Progressive implant migration is the main characteristic of implant instability. A 10-year survival rate of 98% has been reported with the BiCONTACT prosthesis [4].

The introduction of a non-invasive quantitative method for determination of peri-prosthetic bone density has allowed a more detailed analysis of the interaction between the implant and the surrounding bone. Dual energy X-ray absorption (DEXA) bone density measurement permits only planar analysis and therefore measures the bone mineral content (BMC [g]) which with reference to a specified area (cm^2) gives the bone mineral density (BMD [g/cm^2]). The bone mineral content is generally used interchangeably with bone density.

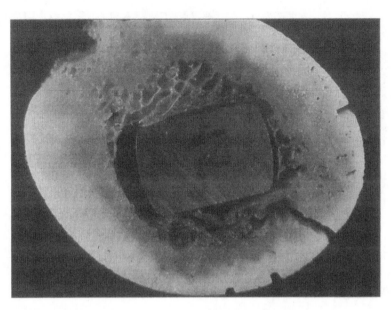

Fig. 8.24. No bony integration occurs in the distal uncoated portion of the BiCONTACT stem. Micromovements are possible here (cut level 18).

Between January 1995 and July 1995, 50 cement-free total hip endoprostheses were implanted and serially assessed by osteodensitometry. In all cases, the BiCONTACT prosthesis was used as the primary implant. The most frequent indication for the operation was idiopathic coxarthrosis. The average age of the patients examined was 57.7 years, with the youngest patient being 29 and the oldest 75.

On the 14th postoperative day ($T = 0$) an X-ray of the hip joint was taken at two levels and bone densitometry was carried out on the operated proximal femur. Further bone density measurements were made on the following day ($T = 1$), after 6 months ($T = 2$) and at 1 year ($T = 3$). At 1 year the hip joint was again X-rayed at two levels. All but one patient regularly attended all the scheduled examinations.

The bone density measurements were made using a DEXA XR 26 bone densitometer. The position of the leg to be examined was controlled by a customised cradle (Fig. 8.25). Reproducibility (and thus accuracy) of bone density measurements with repeated examinations is essential to validate the utility of any device used to measure bone loss or an increased bone formation [32, 57].

To test reproducibility, periprosthetic BMD measurements were performed in a patient with arthrosis of the hip after implantation of a BiCONTACT prosthesis. The measurements were performed on 3 consecutive days with the patient being repositioned for each measurement and the regions of interest being appropriately readjusted (region 0, 1, 7 – see Fig. 8.26). Region 1 (proximal lateral third of prosthesis stem) and Region 7 (prox-

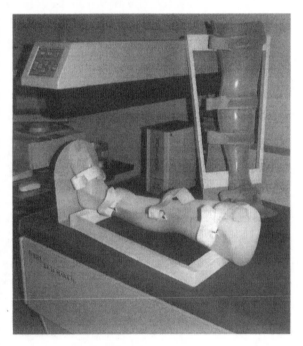

Fig. 8.25. Bone density measuring position "XR 26 bone densitometer". The rail guarantees a rotationally stable position of the leg.

imal medial third of prosthesis stem) corresponded to Gruen zones 1 and 7. The overall region 0 is composed of both regions 1 and 7 (Fig. 8.27). A Plexiglas model with known density parameters was used as a control.

When comparing the BMD coefficients of variation of the model measurements with and without a BiCONTACT stem and the patient measurement

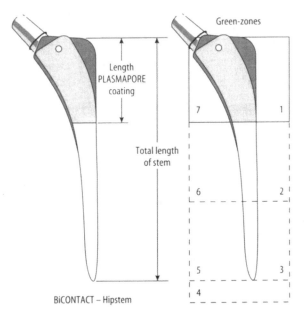

Fig. 8.26. Division of the periprosthetic stem region according to Gruen areas.

after implantation of the stem, it was observed that the BMD coefficient of variation for the model measurement without a prosthesis was the lowest (0.26%), the model measurement with a prosthesis was greater (0.72%), while the patient measurement was the highest (1.04%). These measurements show that the stem prosthesis itself has only a slight influence on the accuracy of the measurement method [28, 29].

The design of the BiCONTACT prosthesis and the distribution of the Plasmapore coating would suggest that the greatest transfer of lead to the bone would be in Gruen zones 1 and 7. The BMD, BMC and area mean values with their standard deviations obtained from the patient group at the four different measurement times are presented in Table 8.2.

In the global region 0, bone density showed an average percentage decrease in the first six months of 18.9% with a further 0.3% decrease in the second 6 months. Qualitatively identical results were obtained for the two regions 1 and 7 (Fig. 8.28). In region 1, the reduction in bone density in the first 6 months was 18.1% compared with 19.4% in region 7. During the second 6 months, bone density increased by 0.5% in region 1 and by 0.7% in region 7. The reduction in periprosthetic bone density in the area of the proximal third of the prosthesis stem

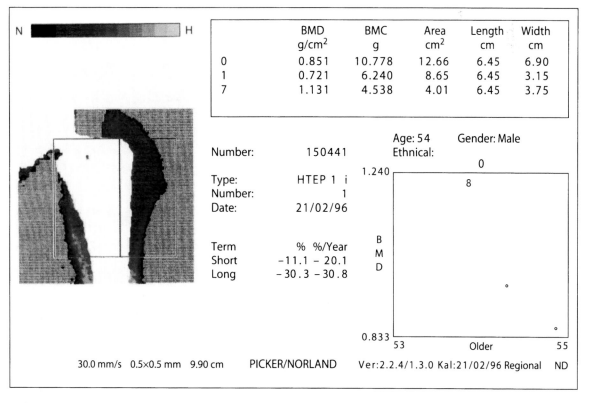

Fig. 8.27. Osteodensitometer measurement area: green zones 1 and 7. The overall region 0 is the sum of the green zones 1 and 7.

Table 8.2. DEXA measurement results of the patient group with BMD, BMC and area mean for the different measurement points [with standard deviations]

		T 0, n = 50	T 1, n = 50	T 2, n = 50	T 3, n = 49
BMD (g/cm²)	Region 0	1.0070 [0.1472]	1.0112 [0.1485]	0.8181 [0.1661]	0.8210 [0.1786]
	Region 1	0.9099 [0.1278]	0.91 [0.1265]	0.7457 [0.1483]	0.7496 [0.1564]
	Region 7	1.1463 [0.2246]	1.1558 [0.2231]	0.9279 [0.2426]	0.9343 [0.2603]
BMC (g)	Region 0	12.6376 [3.0611]	12.6711 [2.9860]	10.2898 [2.8521]	10.3594 [2.7730]
	Region 1	6.5597 [1.8098]	6.5646 [1.7350]	5.5404 [1.8290]	5.6109 [1.8474]
	Region 7	6.0779 [1.7351]	6.1065 [1.7370]	4.7499 [1.4745]	4.7485 [1.3630]
Area mean (cm²)	Region 0	12.486 [2.144]	12.480 [2.126]	12.567 [2.318]	12.671 [2.322]
	Region 1	7.184 [1.580]	7.197 [1.560]	7.377 [1.752]	7.452 [1.741]
	Region 7	5.302 [1.271]	5.283 [1.272]	5.189 [1.329]	5.218 [1.404]

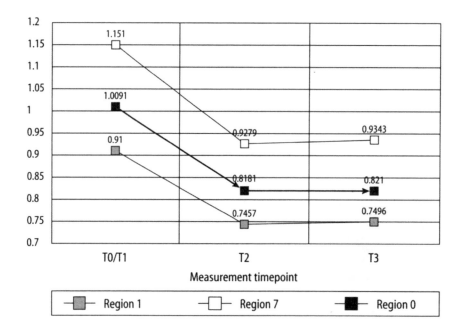

Fig. 8.28. BMD means from the three regions 0, 1 and 7 at 6-monthly intervals during patient measurements on the proximal prosthesis stem.

was significant in the first 6 months. However, further measurements at one year revealed that this remained static and there was no further loss of bone.

A slight increase in periprosthetic bone density was observed immediately after the operation. This can probably be ascribed to impaction of the cancellous bone with the BiCONTACT A- and B-osteoprofilers and to the resultant press-fit implantation.

The fact that the stiffness of implants influences the extent of bone remodelling was demonstrated by Engh et al. [20] and Ang et al. [3]. The stress shielding for stem prostheses with a large stem diameter appeared to be greater and was ascribed to the greater rigidity of these prostheses. The average periprosthetic reduction in the proximal femur in BMD with BiCONTACT stems larger than no. 15 was 29.7%. In contrast, with stem sizes below no. 13 (including the dysplasia stems) the reduction was only 12.6% [28]. This supports the above observations that stem size and rigidity have an influence on bone remodelling.

The critical factor in obtaining reproducibility of the measurements is the exact positioning of the subject to be examined, so that precisely the same region is re-examined during the corresponding repeat measurements. The coefficient of variation obtained from the patient measurement was 1.04% for the entire proximal third of the stem and was therefore greater, as expected, than in the model measurement. However, in the calcar region (region 7) the coefficient of variation was distinctly higher (3.86%), which suggests a lower degree of reproducibility in this region in comparison to region 1. This can almost certainly be ascribed to the morphology of the calcar and the adjacent trochanter minor. The slightest rotational movement of the leg may overlap these bony elements over the metal prosthesis, thus influencing bone density measurements. A wide range of factors can influence the coefficient of variation in different zones and at different times [28, 29].

Bone densitometry cannot replace other important methods of analysing the periprosthetic bone structure, such as histological and radiological examination. Bone densitometry does, however, provide valuable information regarding the bone response to implanted prostheses.

The implantation of a cement-free stem with proximal anchoring produces an interaction between bone mass and implant which occurs primarily in the metaphyseal area of the femur. The influence on the periprosthetic bone structure can be primarily a result of surgical technique, the prosthesis design, the surface composition and bone quality. Periprosthetic bone structure can be affected secondarily by stress shielding and implant loosening. The consequences of implant loosening are well known, whereas the effect of bone remodelling on the durability of prosthetic fixation is less well documented. The development of durable hip endoprostheses may depend in the future on implants which maintain long-term fixation and minimise bone remodelling. Reliable methods of documenting the changes in periprosthetic bone after total hip replacement will then be of particular value.

Summary and Perspective

The fate of a hip joint implant ultimately depends on the interaction between living material – bone – and a prosthesis made out of bioinert material. Ideally, a long-lasting bond will be created between these dissimilar materials. Modifications of material and design require careful biomechanical study and clinical review to determine the impact on long-term results. Critical evaluation of fixation technology and recognition of the results obtained from basic research and clinical experience suggest that there is not one optimal solution, but rather the necessity of tailoring choice of procedure to suit the needs of the individual patient (age, activity profile, etc.). In the majority of cases, this means that the final decision to use a cemented or uncemented prosthesis can only be made intraoperatively. The prosthesis system used should preferably meet all requirements to optimise whichever technique is chosen. Based on a 10-year experience with the BiCONTACT hip prosthesis our feeling is that the system provides this flexibility and fulfils all the criteria of a "state of the art" total hip replacement.

References

1. Åkesson K, Önsten I, Obrant KJ (1994) Periarticular bone in rheumatoid arthritis versus arthrosis. Histomorphometry in 103 hip biopsies. Acta Orthop Scandinavica 65:135–138
2. Alexeef M, Mahomed N, Morsi E, Garbuz D, Gross A (1996) Structural allograft in two-stage revisions for failed septic hip arthroplasty. J Bone Joint Surg 78B(2):213–216
3. Ang KC, Dasde S, Goh IHC, Low SL, Bose K (1997) Periprosthetic bone remodelling after cementless total hip replacement. J Bone Joint Surg Br 79:675–679
4. Asmuth T, Bachmann J, Eingartner C, Feldmann C, aus der Fünten K, Holz F, Hübenthal L, Papp J, Quack, G, Sauer, G (1998) Ergebnisse des zementfrei implantierten BiCONTACT Schaftes – Multicenter Studie mit 553 Fällen. In: Weller S, Braun A, Gekeler R, Volkmann R, Weise K (ed) Das BiCONTACT Hüftendoprothesensystem, Georg Thieme Verlag, Stuttgart, pp 63–74
5. Barrack RL (1995) Economics of revision total hip arthroplasty. Clin Orthop 319:209–214
6. Barrack RL, Mulroy RD Jr., Harris WH (1992) Improved cementing techniques and femoral component loosening in young patients with hip arthroplasty. A 12-year radiographic review. J Bone Joint Surg 74B(3):385–389
7. Blömer W, Ungethüm M (1992) Überlegungen zum Pfannendesign. Sphärisch oder konisch? Gewinde selbstschneidend oder geschnitten. In: Hipp E, Gradinger R, Ascherl R (ed) Die zementlose Hüftprothese. Demeter
8. Bobyn JD, Pilliar RM, Cameron HU, Weatherly GC (1980) The optimum pore size for the fixation of porous surfaced metal implants by the ingrowth of bone. Clin Orthop 150:263–270
9. Bülow JUG, Scheller G, Arnold P, Synatschke M, Jani L (1996) Uncemented total hip replacement and tight pain. Int Orthop 20:65–69

10. Cameron HU, Pilliar RM, Macnab J (1973) The effect of movement on the bonding of porous metal to bone. J Biomed Mater Res 7:301–311

11. Chmell MJ, Scott RD, Thomas WH, Sledge CB (1997) Total hip arthroplasty with cement for juvenile rheumatoid arthrotis. Results at a minimum of ten years in patients less than thirty years old. J Bone Joint Surg 79A:44–52

12. Cook SD, Thomas KA, Kay SF, Jarcho M (1988) Hydroxylapatite-Coated Porous Titanium for Use as an Orthopaedic Biologic Attachment System. Clin Orthop 230:303–312

13. Cordero J, Munuera L, Folgueira MD (1994). Influence of metal implants on infection. An experimental study in rabbits. J Bone Joint Surg 76 B(5):717–720

14. David A, Eitenmüller J, Muhr G, Pommer A, Bär HF, Ostermann PAW, Schildhauer, TA (1995) Mechanical and histological evaluation of hydroxyapatite-coated, titanium-coated and gritblasted surfaces under weight bearing conditions. Arch Orthop Trauma Surg 114:112–118

15. David A, Lewandrowski KU, Eitenmüller J, Muhr G, Pommer A, Bär HF, Ostermann, PAW (1996) Interlocking strength in hydroxyapatite- and titanium-coated implants under weightbearing conditions: A biomechanical and histologic study. Orthopaedics International Edition 4, 3:209–218

16. Dorey F, Amstutz HC (1986) Survivorship Analysis in the evaluating of joint replacement. J Arthroplasty 1:63–69

17. Duncan CP, Masri BA (1994) The role of antibiotic-loaded cement in the treatment of an infection after a hip replacement. J Bone Joint Surg 76A:1742–1751

18. Eckert H (1988) Das zementlose Hüftendoprothesensystem Zweymüller-Endler, kurz- und mittelfristige Ergebnisse. MD thesis, University of München

19. Eingartner C, Volkmann R, Kümmel K, Weller S (1997) Niedrige Lockerungsrate einer zementierten Geradschaftprothese im längerfristigen Verlauf. Swiss Surg 2:49–54

20. Engh CA, Bobyn JD, Glassmann AH, (1987) Porous-coated hip replacenent. J Bone Joint Surg Br 69:45–55

21. Engh CA, Massin P, Suthers KE (1990) Roentgenographic assessment of the biologic fixation of porous-surfaced femoral components. Clin Orthop 257:107–128

22. Engh CA, Hooten JP, Zettl-Schaffer KF, Ghaffarpour M, Mc Gover TF, Macalino GE (1994) Porous-coated total hip replacement. Clin Orthop 298:89–96

23. Engh CA Jr, Culpepper WJ 2nd, Engh CA (1997) Long-term results of use of the anatomic medullary locking prosthesis in total hip arthroplasty. J Bone Joint Surg Am 79(2):177–184

24. Fink U (1996) PLASMAPORE: A plasma-sprayed microporous Titanium coating to improve the long term stability. In: Naivard D, Merle M, Delagoutte JP, Louis JP, Sedel L (ed): Actualités en Biomatériaux 111:97–104

25. Frost HM (1988) Vital biomechanics, proposed general concepts for skeletal adaptations to mechanical usage. Calcif Tissue Int 42:145–156

26. Garvin KL, Hanssen AD (1995) Current concepts review. Infection after total hip arthroplasty. Past, present and future. J Bone Joint Surg 77A:1576–1588

27. Geesink RG, Hoefnagels NH (1995) Six-year results of hydroxyapatite-coated total hip replacement. J Bone Surg Br 77(4):534–547

28. Gellrich JC (1998) Osteodensiometrische und radiologische Beurteilung zum Einheilungsverhalten zementfreier Hüftendoprothesen (BiCONTACT). MD thesis, University of Heidelberg

29. Gellrich JC, Braun A, Gross U (1998) Histologische und osteodensitometrische Untersuchungen periprothetischer Knochenreaktionen am zementfrei implantierten BiCONTACT-Schaft. In: Weller S, Braun A, Gekeler R, Volkmann R, Weise K (ed) Das BiCONTACT Hüftendoprothesensystem, Georg Thieme Verlag, Stuttgart, pp 189–200

30. Gross U (1985) Verbundvorhaben Verbesserung der Langzeitstabilität von Endoprothesen: Messung biologischer Wirkungsgrößen am Interface oberflächenaktiver Implantatmaterialien. Förderkennzeichen 01 VT 8603 Bundesministerium für Forschung und Technologie

31. Gustillo RB, Burnham WH (1982) Long-term results of total hip arthroplasty in young patients. In: The Hip. Proceedings of the Tenth Open Scientific Meeting of the Hip Society. St. Louis, C. V. Mosby, pp. 27–33

32. Hagemann JE (1990) Knochendichtemessung. Eigenverlag Picker International GmbH Picker aktuell 15:43–45

33. Hanssen AD, Osmon DR, Nelson CL (1996) Prevention of deep periprosthetic joint infection. J Bone Joint Surg 78A:458–471

34. Harris WH, Davies JP (1988) Modern use of modern cement for total hip replacement. Clin Orthop 19:581–589

35. Helfen M, Malzer U, Peters P, Griss P, Himmelmann G, Weber E (1993) Zementfreie Pfanne und zementierter Schaft – Konzept einer "Hybrid-Lösung" sowie Ergebnisse einer drei- bis sechsjährigen klinischen Erfahrung. Z Orthop 131:578–584

36. Herberts P, Ahnfelt L, Malchau H, Strömberg C, Andersson GBJ (1989) Multicenter clinical trials and their value in assessing total joint arthroplasty. Clin Orthop 249:48–55

37. Hozack WJ, Rothmann RH, Booth RE Jr, Balderston RA, Cohn JC, Pickens GT (1990) Survivorship analysis of 1,041 Charnley total hip arthroplasties. J Arthroplasty 5:41–47

38. Jasty M, Maloney WJ, Bragdon CR, Haire T, Harris WH (1990) Histomorphological studies of the long-term skeletal responses to well fixed cemented femoral components. J Bone Joint Surg 72A:1220–1229

39. Joshi AB, Porter ML, Trail IA, Hunt LP, Murphy JC, Hardinge K (1993) Long-term results of Charnley low-friction arthroplasty in young patients. J Bone Joint Surg 75B(4):616–623

40. Kiratli BJ, Heiner JP, Mc Beath AA, Wilson MA (1992) Determination of bone mineral density by dual X-ray absorptiometry in patients with uncemented total hip arthroplasty. J Orthop Res 10:836–844

41. Korovessis P, Repanti M (1994) Evolution of aggressive granulomatous periprosthetic lesions in cemented hip arthroplasties. Clin Orthop 155–161

42. MacKenzie JR, Kelley SS, Johnston RC (1996) Total hip replacement for coxarthrosis secondary to congenital dysplasia and dislocation of the hip. Long-term results. J Bone Joint Surg 78A:55–61

43. Mallory TH, Head WC, Lombardi jr AV, Emerson jr RH, Eberle RW, Mitchell MB (1996) Clinical and radiographic outcome of a cementless, titanium, plasma-coated total hip arthroplasty femoral component. Justification for continuance of use. J Arthroplasty 11(6):653–660

44. Marston RA, Cobb AG, Bentley G (1996) Stanmore compared with Charnley total hip replacement. A prospective study of 413 hip arthroplasties. J Bone Joint Surg 78B(2):178–184

45. McCoy TH, Salvati EA, Ranawat CS, Wilson PD Jr. (1988) A fifteen-year follow-up study of one hundred Charnley low-friction arthroplasties. Clin Orthop 19:467–476

46. Mulroy RD Jr., Harris WH (1990) The effect of improved cementing techniques on component loosening in total hip replacement. An 11-year radiographic review. J Bone Joint Surg 72B(5):757–760

47. Mulroy WF, Harris WH (1996) Revision total hip arthroplasty with use of so-called second-generation cementing techniques for aseptic loosening of the femoral component. A fifteen-year average follow-up study. J Bone Joint Surg 78A:325–330

48. Neumann L, Freund KG, Sorensen KH (1996) Total hip arthroplasty with the Charnley prosthesis in patients fifty-

five years old and less. Fifteen to twenty-one-year results. J Bone Joint Surg 78A:73–79

49. Okamoto T, Inao S, Gototh E, Ando M (1997) Primary Charnley total hip arthroplasty for congenital dysplasia: effect of improved techniques of cementing. J Bone Joint Surg 79B(1):83–86

50. Ottenbach A, Breitenfelder J (1996) Mittelfristige Ergebnisse der zementlosen Hüftgelenktotalendoprothetik: BiContact-Modell versus Mittelmeier-Hüfte. Orthopädische Praxis 92 (4):224–227

51. Pitto RP, Böhner J, Hofmeister V (1997) Einflußgrößen der Primärstabilität acetabulärer Komponenten. Eine In-vitro-Studie. Biomed, Technik 42:363–368

52. Puhl W (ed) (1997): Performance of the Wear Couple BIOLOX forte. In: Hip Arthroplasty. Enke, Stuttgart

53. Refior HJ (ed) (1987) Zementfreie Implantation von Hüftgelenksendoprothesen – Standortbestimmung und Tendenzen. Thieme, Stuttgart, New York

54. Roesler H (1997) The history of some fundamental concepts in bone biomechanics. J Biomechanics 20:1025–1034

55. Smith SE; Harris WH (1997) Total Hip Arthroplasty Performed with Insertion of the Femoral Component with Cement and the Acetabular Component without Cement. J Bone Joint Surg 79A:1827–1833

56. Sochart DH, Porter ML (1997) Long-term results of total hip replacement in young patients who had ankylosing spondylitis. J Bone Joint Surg 79–A:1181–1189

57. Spitz J, Stoecker M, Clemenz N, Kempers B, Fischer M (1990) Vergleichende Messung des Knochenmineralgehalts mit DPA – Erste klinische Erfahrungen. Fortschr Röntgenstr. 152:340–344

58. Sumner DR, Turner TM, Urban RM, Galante JO (1992) Remodelling and ingrowth of bone at two years in a canine cementless total hip arthroplasty model. J Bone Joint Surg 74A:239–250

59. Torchia ME, Klassen RA, Bianco AJ (1996) Total hip arthroplasty with cement in patients less than twenty years old. Long-term results. J Bone Joint Surg 78A:995–1003

60. Weller S, Volkmann R (1994) Das Bicontact-Hüftendoprothesen-System. Thieme, Stuttgart 1994

61. Weller S (1997) "Cement or Cementless Fixation" – an individual decision in Total Hip Arthroplasty. International Orthop 11. Implant Special, Springer 1997

62. Widmer KH, Zurfluh B, Morscher EW (1997) Kontaktfläche und Druckbelastung im Implantat-Knochen-Interface bei Press-Fit Hüftpfannen im Vergleich zum natürlichen Hüftgelenk. Orthopädie 26:181–189

63. Willert HG (1996) Clinical relevance of wear particles to osteolysis and loosening of hip endoprostheses. In: Puhl W (ed): Die Keramikpaarung BIOLOX in der Hüftendoprothetik. Enke, Stuttgart

64. Winkelmann HP, Gersmann M, Gunselmann M (1996) Die operative Behandlung von hüftgelenksnahen Femurfrakturen beim alten Menschen im Wandel der letzten 20 Jahre. Akt Traumatol 26:73–78

65. Winkler-Gniewek W, Stallforth H, Ungethüm M (1988) Die Plasmapore-Beschichtung von Gelenkendoprothesen – ein neues Konzept. In: Friedebold G (ed) Oberflächenkonstruierte Prothesen aus technischer und medizinischer Sicht. DMV, Berlin

66. Winkler-Gniewek W (1989) Die Plasmapore-Beschichtung für die zementlose Verankerung von Gelenkendoprothesen. Aesculap Wissenschaftliche Information im Selbstverlag

67. Wolff J (1892) Das Gesetz der Transformation der Knochen. Hirschwald, Berlin

68. Wroblewski MB (1986) 15–21-year results of the Charnley low-friction arthroplasty. Clin Orthop 211:30–35

69. Wroblewski MB, Siney PD (1993) Charnley low-friction arthroplasty of the hip. Long-term results. Clin Orthop 292:191–201

Section V

Articular Interface

9. Polyethylene as a Bearing Surface

J.E. Parr, W. Haggard and H.H. Trieu

The Issue of Polyethylene Wear

Ultra-high molecular-weight polyethylene (UHMWPE) is the most commonly used bearing material in total joint replacement. Wear of UHMWPE is a serious clinical problem that limits the longevity of orthopaedic implants. Excessive wear may lead to gross mechanical failure such as fracture and disassociation [3] and the release of particulate wear debris may induce biological responses that cause implant loosening [4, 5].

Researchers have documented excessive wear in retrieved tibial, patellar and acetabular components of joint replacements. The degree of wear reported often depends upon factors unrelated to the polyethylene quality such as patient age [6–9], activity level [10], body weight [9, 11–13] implantation time [14, 15] component alignment, component thickness [16, 17] and articular geometry [16–18]. However, control of polyethylene quality is essential for the improvement of wear resistance. Maintaining the original properties of polyethylene is also very important to its in-vivo performance. Therefore, any potential adverse effects on polyethylene that may be caused by processing, manufacturing or sterilisation should be avoided or minimised.

Raw Material and Processing

Lot-controlled medical-grade UHMWPE in the form of an extruded bar is the most common type of starting material for many companies who require that this material pass internal specifications which meet or in many cases *exceed* the industry standard (ASTM F648). The molecular weight (measured by relative solution viscosity), trace element composition, extraneous material and powder particle size are characterised and the powder is used only if it passes strict internal specifications.

If properly controlled, both extrusion or compression-moulding are acceptable processing methods. Currently, most companies produce UHMWPE components by machining or solid-phase forming extruded raw material. Proper fusion of the resin powder is ensured by carefully controlling the extrusion rate and die temperature. Ultrasonic and optical inspection of thin slices of the raw material ensure that the probability of fusion defects in the raw material is minimised.

An additional advantage of the extrusion process is that it is a closed process. The powder is fed from its shipping container directly to the extrusion die in a closed system. This minimises the possibility of introducing particulate contamination during extrusion. After extrusion, the raw material is annealed to remove residual stresses and to enhance dimensional stability. Hot stamping of UHMWPE components is to be avoided since this process has been shown to lead to premature delamination.

Mechanical Properties

The mechanical properties of the UHMWPE have been well characterised and demonstrate its high quality and consistency. Mechanical property data is inherently variable and requires multiple samples of at least three specimens (preferably five specimens) per sample to be statistically meaningful. No data should be presented without reporting the statistical information necessary for a complete understanding of its relevance. Extruded and annealed UHMWPE

Table 9.1. Typical mechanical properties of UHMWPE (Wright Medical Technology, Inc.)

Mechanical property	ASTM method	Specimen/condition	Mean μ	Standard deviation δ	ASTM F648 specification
Tensile yield strength (psi)	D638	Type IV 2 in per min	3251	96	2800 min
Ultimate tensile strength (psi)	D638	Type IV 2 in per min	5709	621	4000 min
Ultimate tensile elongation (%)	D638	Type IV 2 in per min	347	32	200 min
Izod impact strength (ft–lbf/in^2)	D256	Type A Double 15° notch	No break	–	20 min
Deformation under load (%)	D621	23°C 1000 psi	0.92	0.11	2 max
Hardness	D2240	Shore D	68.7	0.97	60 min

Note: 1 lbf/in^2 (psi) = 6.9 kPa.

can consistently exceed the mechanical property requirements of ASTM F648 (Table 9.1).

Oxidative Degradation of UHMWPE

Gamma radiation has been a common sterilisation method for UHMWPE used in total joint replacement. The products are sterilised by gamma radiation from a cobalt 60 source. It is well known that gamma radiation induces various chemical changes in plastics which lead to oxidation, and several studies have recently discussed the oxidation of UHMWPE following radiation and ageing [19–23]. In 1984 and 1987, Eyerer and co-workers [24, 25] reported oxidation in several acetabular components. Li et al. suggested that oxidation of UHMWPE continues for long periods of time after gamma radiation. Saum [21] reported subsurface oxidation which remained significant to 2 mm below the surface. Oxidation as deep as 3 mm into the samples was also found by Rimnac and co-workers [22]. Trieu and Paxson [26] have recently demonstrated an oxidised surface layer as thick as 6 mm in UHMWPE components.

The common understanding of the oxidation mechanism is as follows: UHMWPE initially consists of extremely long molecular chains, which makes it an excellent abrasion-resistant material. Sterilisation by gamma radiation causes chain scission by breaking chemical bonds and creates reactive free radicals. Oxygen diffuses into the material and reacts with free radicals to cause oxidation, which leads to much shorter molecular chains. As a result, the original properties of polyethylene, including abrasion resistance, change significantly. Preliminary data indicate that long-term oxidative degradation can alter the performance of polyethylene in total joint replacement, especially its resistance to fatigue wear. This can cause pitting and delamination. The effect of oxidation on polyethylene wear will be discussed later in this technical report.

The Oxidised Surface Layer in UHMWPE Components

The authors have been actively investigating the effect of sterilisation on polyethylene [26–29]. A polishing technique was developed to document the oxidised surface layer in UHMWPE products that had been sterilised by gamma radiation and aged on the shelf for various durations [26]. The effect of postradiation ageing on the oxidised surface was also investigated using infrared (IR) microscopy, differential scanning calorimetry (DSC), density measurement, hardness testing and tensile testing [27–29].

Figure 9.1 shows the cross-sections of polyethylene components that have been stored on the shelf following sterilisation by gamma radiation. The cross-sections reveal a surface layer and a core region separated by a boundary line that is located at a consistent depth below the contoured surface of the samples. The IR data indicate that the surface layer has been oxidised extensively while minimal oxidation was detected in the core. Under the same polishing conditions, the surface layer became much smoother than the core region, most probably as a

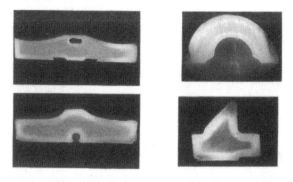

Fig. 9.1. Cross-sections of UHMWPE components showing an oxidised surface layer and a core region with minimal oxidation.

result of the difference in abrasion resistance between the surface and the core. It is believed that the original abrasion resistance of the surface layer altered as the polyethylene undergoes oxidation. In fact, Fisher and co-workers [30] have recently reported a three-fold increase in the wear factor of UHMWPE following radiation and ageing compared to the non-irradiated material.

The oxidation level within a tibial component that has been shelf-aged for 87 months post radiation is shown in Fig. 9.2. Maximum oxidation occurs approximately 1 to 2 mm below the surface, and the oxidation level decreases as the core is approached. Thickness of this oxidised surface layer increases with increasing ageing time, as shown in Fig. 9.3. The thickness increases rapidly within the first 2 years and appears to level off at approximately 5 to 6 mm. However, the level of oxidation in the surface layer continues to increase for several years. The visual difference between the material on the surface layer and that in the core is more obvious for the samples with longer ageing time. Density of the surface layer was also found to increase upon ageing as the material became more crystalline. The increase in density that is associated with oxidation has been reported by Rimnac et al. [22–23]. The difference in hardness between the surface layer and the core increases with ageing of the samples. The data indicate that not only does the oxidised surface layer expand in thickness but it also becomes more oxidised upon ageing. The oxidisation of UHMWPE components appears to be a diffusion-limited process. With the initial irradiation of the samples scission occurred with the formation of free radicals [30]. With ageing, oxygen continuously diffused into

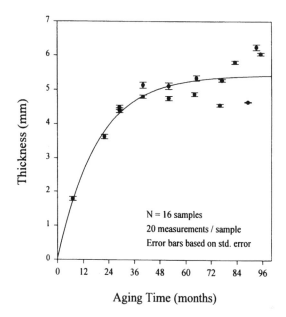

Fig. 9.3. Effect of post-radiation ageing time on thickness of the oxidised surface layer.

the material and reacted with free radicals near the surface.. Oxygen also penetrated deeper into the material to induce more oxidation with time, as shown in Fig. 9.3. As a result, the oxidised surface layer became more oxidised and thickened with time.

Effects of Sterilisation Methods on UHMWPE Properties

The two sterilisation methods that are commonly used for medical plastics are gamma radiation and ethylene oxide. The first method sterilises products using radiation of gamma rays from a cobalt-60 source. As discussed earlier, gamma radiation can lead to extensive oxidation in polyethylene. The second method uses a gas sterilant, ethylene oxide (EtO), to sterilise the products. EtO sterilisation is commonly used for products that are sensitive to the heat of steam sterilisation or materials that may be deteriorated by radiation sterilisation.

Figure 9.4 is a comparison of the typical oxidation levels of polyethylene components that were sterilised by EtO or gamma radiation, and aged on the shelf for 55 and 53 months, respectively. Minimal oxidation was detected for the components sterilised by EtO while significant oxidation was found in the components sterilised by gamma radiation. Since the components were manufactured from different lots of bar stock, the material changes due to oxidation in the surface layer were determined by comparison

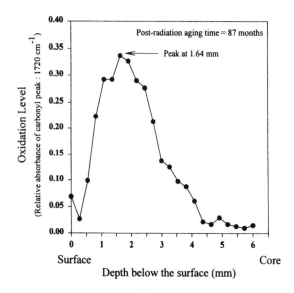

Fig. 9.2. Oxidation profile of a UHMWPE tibial component.

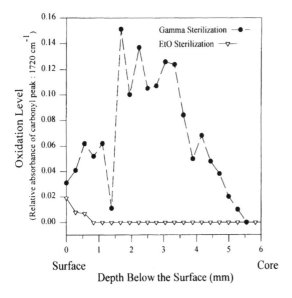

Fig. 9.4. Typical oxidation profiles from the surface to the core of polyethylene tibial components. The components were sterilised by EtO gas and gamma radiation and stored on the shelf for 55 and 53 months, respectively.

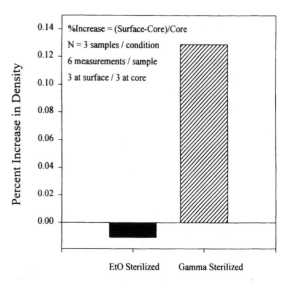

UHMWPE Condition

Fig. 9.6. Percentage increase in density of the surface layer compared to the core region.

with the core region. As shown in Fig. 9.5, a large increase in crystallinity of the surface layer was found in the components in the components sterilised by gamma radiation but not in the ones sterilised by EtO. The increase in crystallinity indicates a substantial change in polyethylene morphology as a result of oxidation. Similarly, Fig. 9.6 reveals an increase in density of the oxidised surface

layer as the material became more crystalline in the case of gamma sterilisation. There is a very small difference in density between the surface and the core for EtO sterilised products, which indicates minimal changes of the surface layer.

The chemical effects of radiation on polyethylene not only lead to changes in the morphology and physical properties but also result in significant changes of mechanical properties. Figure 9.7 reveals that an appreciable difference in hardness (Shore D)

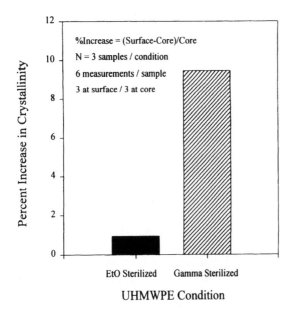

Fig. 9.5. Percentage increase in crystallinity of the surface layer compared to the core region.

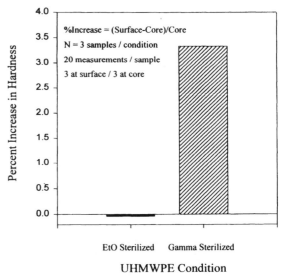

Fig. 9.7. Percentage increase in hardness of the surface layer compared to the core region.

occurs between the surface layer and the core for gamma sterilisation, while there is virtually no difference in the case of EtO sterilisation. Ultimate elongation, which indicates the material ductility, is an important property that is related to the excellent toughness and outstanding wear resistance of UHMWPE.

Elongation of UHMWPE was found to be very sensitive to oxidation as shown in Fig. 9.8. There is only a small difference in elongation between the surface and the core of a polyethylene component sterilised by EtO and aged for 55 months. For the components sterilised by gamma radiation and aged for 53 months, the elongation is approximately 30% lower for the surface than the core. The reduction in elongation of the surface layer becomes larger as oxidation progresses with ageing. As shown in Fig. 9.9, minimal reduction in toughness was observed for UHMWPE sterilised by EtO, while extensive reduction in toughness was found in the case of gamma sterilisation. Similar to elongation, the reduction in toughness of the surface layer is more severe upon ageing. This indicates an increase in surface embrittlement that is caused by oxidation.

How Effective is Inert-gas Packaging?

Gamma radiation causes polyethylene to become reactive due to the formation of free radicals, which later react with oxygen to cause oxidation. The type of polyethylene currently available for orthopaedic

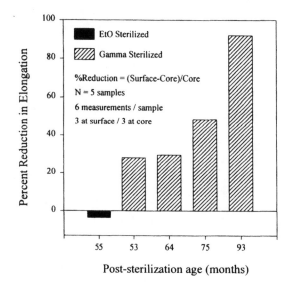

Fig. 9.8. Percentage reduction in elongation of the surface layer compared to the core region.

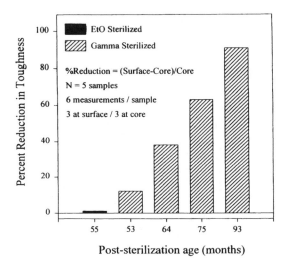

Fig. 9.9. Percentage reduction in toughness of the surface layer compared to the core region.

implants, whether it has medium or high crystallinity, is prone to oxidation during and following gamma radiation. Some manufacturers have recently attempted to prevent oxidation by sterilising polyethylene in an inert or oxygen-free environment such as argon or nitrogen. This may help to reduce the initial oxidation that occurs during sterilisation, but it cannot eliminate oxidation due to the presence of dissolved oxygen in polyethylene. Ries et al. [31] have recently shown that sterilisation in inert gas does not prevent free radicals from causing oxidation for this reason. Several recent studies have shown that oxidation of gamma-irradiated products is taking place over a long period of time [20–23, 26, 27, 29] because long-lived free radicals exist in polyethylene as a result of reduced mobility within crystalline regions [32]. In fact, research at Wright Medical Technology has shown that the majority of oxidation occurs during post-radiation ageing and not during the sterilisation process [26, 27, 29]. Since most plastic packaging materials are poor oxygen barriers in the long term, the initial inert environment is expected to vanish as oxygen continuously permeates into the package after sterilisation. Polyethylene is consequently subjected to oxidation during the critical ageing period. Furthermore, in-vivo oxidation is a potential concern for irradiated UHMWPE. Therefore, the inert-gas packaging approach does not appear as effective as EtO sterilisation in prevention of polyethylene oxidation.

Effects of Sterilisation Methods on the Wear Performance of UHMWPE

Wear testing was performed using both gamma radiation and EtO gas sterilised 20mm thick tibial inserts machined from the same GUR415 UHMWPE bar stock. More than 48 months had elapsed since the components were sterilised and stored on the shelf. A ball-on-flat sliding test was chosen as the wear model. The use of ball-on-flat wear models has been employed by Walker et al. and was observed to produce fatigue failure (i.e. delamination) in the polyethylene which was similar to that seen in retrievals [33–40]. Polished balls with a diameter of 32 mm were loaded against the plastic with a force of 2000 N. In addition the ball was oscillated along a 12.7-mm track at 1 Hz. Filtered calf serum was used as the lubricant. Sodium azide was used to prevent bacterial decay of the serum, and distilled water was added to replace water lost due to evaporation.

Delamination failures like the one shown in Fig. 9.10 occurred with the gamma sterilised/shelf-aged specimens ($n = 6$) after an average of 587 070 cycles as depicted in Fig. 9.12. The fatigue failures

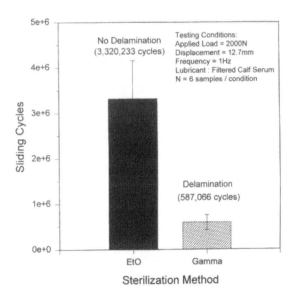

Fig. 9.12. Results of the ball-on-flat sliding wear test.

of these specimens is believed to be caused by the reduction in toughness or increase in brittleness of the surface layer due to oxidation. The typical EtO sterilised/shelf-aged wear specimen shown in Fig. 9.11 reveals only a depression that is caused by the normal creep behaviour of UHMWPE. There was no delamination observed with the EtO-sterilised/shelf-aged wear specimens($n = 6$) after an average of 3.3 million cycles (Fig. 9.12). The excellent resistance to fatigue failure of EtO-sterilised specimens is attributed to the minimal effects that EtO sterilisation has on UHMWPE properties.

Why is Ethylene Oxide (EtO) Sterilisation Preferred?

The three main factors that collectively lead to excessive oxidation in shelf-aged UHMWPE components are: (1) free radicals induced by gamma radiation; (2) oxygen from the environment; and (3) time for oxygen to diffuse into the polyethylene. Oxidation can be minimised by eliminating one of the three factors. However, since in-vivo oxidation is also a potential concern for irradiated UHMWPE, elimination of reactive free radicals is the best approach. Our research has demonstrated that this can be achieved using ethylene oxide (EtO) sterilisation. As shown in Fig. 9.13, the EtO-sterilised component does not have the oxidised surface layer that is commonly found in gamma-sterilised components (Fig. 9.14) with a similar post-sterilisation age (greater than 4 years). With a commitment to

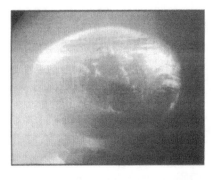

Fig. 9.10. Gamma-sterilised, shelf-aged water test specimens after 540 000 sliding cycles.

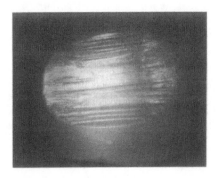

Fig. 9.11. EtO-sterilised, shelf-aged wear test specimen after 5.1 million sliding cycles.

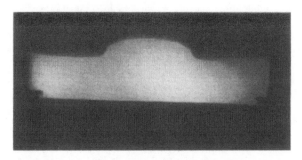

Fig. 9.13. A cross-section of EtO-sterilised/shelf-aged UHMWPE tibial components.

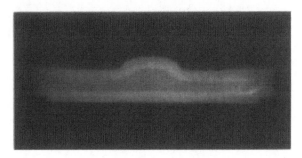

Fig. 9.14. A typical cross-section of gamma-sterilised/shelf-aged UHMWPE tibial components.

improve the wear resistance of polyethylene, companies such as Wright Medical Technology now sterilise their polyethylene products by EtO to minimise oxidation.

Conclusion

Increasing focus on polyethylene wear factors has prompted various attempts to improve the wear resistance of UHMWPE. One of the primary factors that influence the polyethylene wear performance is the material quality itself. Recognising this, companies have optimised their polyethylene by careful raw resin selection, optimising extrusion, and enhancing manufacturing. The excellent quality and properties (e.g. wear and fatigue resistance) of the original polyethylene products are well preserved by sterilising with ethylene oxide gas instead of gamma radiation, which is well known to cause oxidative degradation.

References

1. Lombardi, A-V Jr, Engh GA, Volz RG, Albrigo JL, Brainard BJ. Fracture/dissassociation of the polyethylene in metal-backed patellar components in total knee arthroplasty. J Bone Joint Surg 1988;70-A (6):675–679.

2. Stulberg SD, Stulberg BN, Harnati Y, Tsao A. Failure mechanisms of metal-backed patellar components. Clin Orthop 1988;236:88–105.

3. Wright TM, Rimnac CM, Stulberg SD et al. Wear of polyethylene in total joint replacement: observations from retrieved PCA knee implants. Clin Orthop 1992;276:126–134.

4. Peters PC, Engh GA, Dwyer KA, Vinh TN. Osteolysis after total knee arthroplasty without cement. J Bone Joint Surg 1992;74A(7):864–876.

5. Santavirta S, Konttinen YT, Hoikka V, Eskola A. Immunopathological response to loose cementless acetabular components. J Bone Joint Surg 1991;73B(I):38–42.

6. Clarke IC. Titanium alloy alumina ceramics and UHMWPE use in total joint replacemen. In: SM Lee (ed.) Advances in biomaterials. Lancaster, PA, Technomic Pub, 1987; 217–232.

7. Halley, DK and Wroblewski BM. Long-term results of low-friction arthroplasty in patients 30 years of age or younger. Clin Orthop 1986;211:43–50.

8. Moreland JR, Jinnah R. Fracture of a Charnley acetabular component from polyethlylene wear. Clin Orthop 1986; 207:94–96.

9. Bartel D, Bicknell VL, Wright TM. The effect of conformity thickness and material on stresses on ultra-high molecular weight components in total joint replacement. J Bone Joint Surg 1986;68A(7):1041–1051.

10. Dowson D, Wallbridge NC. Laboratory wear tests and clinical observations of the penetration of femoral heads into acetabular cups in total replacement hip joints 1: Charnley prosthesis with polytetrafluoroethylene acetabular cups. Wear 1985;104:203–221.

11. Salvati EA, Wilson PD. A ten-year follow-up of our first one hundred consecutive Charnley total hip replacements. J Bone Joint Surg 1981;63A(5):753–767.

12. Wright TM, Burstein AH, Bartel DL. Retrieval analysis of total joint replacements: A six-year experience. Proceedings of the Second Annual Symposium on Corrosion and Degradation of Implant Materials, Philadelphia. ASTM, 1985;415–429.

13. Salvati EA, Wright TM, Burstein AH, Bartel DL. Fracture of polyethylene acetabular cups J Bone Joint Surg 1979;61A(8): 1239–1242.

14. Yaniamuro T. Advances in clinical use of artificial joint of the hip and knee In: LR Rubin (ed.) Biomaterials in reconstructive surgery. St Louis: CV Mosby Co, 1993; 339–377.

15. Wroblewski BM. Direction and rate of socket wear in Charnley low friction arthroplasty. J Bone Joint Surg 1985;67B(5):757–761.

16. BarteL DL, Burstein AH, Toda MD, Edwards DL. The effect of conformity and plastic thickness on contact stresses in metal-backed plastic implants. J Biomech Eng 1985;107:193.

17. Collier JP, Mayor MB, Surprenant VA, Suprenant HP Dauphinais LA, Jensen RE. The biological problems of polyethylene as a bearing surface Clin Orthop 1990;261:107.

18. Bloebaum RD, Nelson K,- Dorr LD, Hoffman AA, Lyman DJ. Investigation of early delamination observed in retrieved heat treated tibial inserts Clin Orthop 1991;269:120.

19. Streichcr RM. Ionizing irradiation for sterilization and modification of high molecular weight polyethylenes. Plast Rubber Proc Appl 1988;10:221–229.

20. Li S, Saum KA, Collier JP, Kasprazak D. Oxidation of UMHWPE over long time periods. Trans Soc Biomater 1994;17:425.

21. Saun KA. Oxidation vs depth and time for polyethylene-gamma sterilized in air. Trans ORS 1994;19:174:130.

22. Rimnac CM. Klcin RW, Khanna N, Weintraub JT. Post-irradiation aging of ultra high molecular weight polyethylene. Trans Soc Biomater 1993;16:328.

23. Rimnac CM Klein RW, Betts F, Wright TM. Post-irradiation aging of ultra high molecular weight polyethylene J Bone Joint Surg 1994;76A(7):1052–1056.

24. Eyerer P, Ke YC. Properties changes of UHMW polyethylene hip cup endoprostheses J Biol Mater Res 1984;18:1137–1151.

25. Eyerer P, Kurth NM, McKellup HA, Mittlmeier T. Characterization of UHMWPE hip cups on joint simulators. J Biol Mater Res 1987;21:275–291.

26. Trieu HH, Paxson RD. The oxidized surface layer in shelf-aged UHMWPE implants. Trans Orth 1995;758.

27. Trieu HH, Avent R, Paxson RD. Effect of sterilisation on shelf-aged UHMWPE tibial inserts. Trans Soc Biomat 1995;18:109.

28. Trieu HH, Avent R. Effect of sterilisation on UHMWPE implants. Accepted for the SecondAnnual Combined Orthopaedic Research Societies Meeting in 1995.

29. Fisher J, Hailey JL, Chan KL, Shaw D, Stone M. The effect of ageing following irradiation on the wear of UHMWPE. Trans ORS 1995;20:120.

30. Ries M, Rose R, Greer J, Weaver K, Sauer W, Beals N. Sterilisation induced effects on UHMWPE performance. Trans ORS 1995;20:757.

31. Chapiro A. Tech Dev Prospects Steril Ioniz- Radiat Int Conf 1974; 367–374.

32. Blunn GW, Joshi A, Engelbrecht E, Lilley PA, Harding K, Walker PS. A retrieval and in-vitro study of degradation of ultra-high molecular weight polyethylene total knee replacements. Fourth World Biomaterials Conference 1992; 276

33. Blunn GW Joshi AB, Walker PS. Performance of ultra-high molecular weight polyethylene in knee replacement. Trans ORS 1993;18:500.

34. Walker PS, Blunn GW, Joshi AB, Sathasivam S. Modulation of delamination by surface wear in total knees. Trans ORS 1993;18:499.

35. Blunn GW Joshi A, Hardinge K, Engelbrecht E, Walker PS. The effect of bearing conformity on the wear of polyethylene tibial components. Trans ORS 1992;17:357.

36. Blunn GW, Walker PS, Joshi A, Hardinge K. The dominance of cyclic sliding in producing wear in total knee replacements. Clin Orthop 1991;273:253–260.

37. Walker PS, Salvati E. The measurement and effects of friction and wear in artificial hip joints J Biomed Mater Res Symp 1973;4:327–342.

38. Kilgus DJ, Moreland JR, Finerman AM, Funahashi TT, Tipton JS. Catastrophic wear of tibial polyethylene insets. Clin Orthop 1991;273:223–231.

39. Landy MM, Walker PS. Wear of ultra-high-molecular-weight polyethylene components of 90 retrieved knee prostheses. J Arthroplasty 1988;3:S73–S84.

10. The Metal/Polyethylene Interface

J.L. Tipper, A.A. Besong, H. Minakawa, M.H. Stone,
B.M. Wroblewski, E. Ingham and J. Fisher

Introduction

Total hip replacements have been used for over 30 years with considerable success. Approximately 50,000 hip joints are replaced each year in the UK, and world-wide that figure rises to approximately 800,000. Today the most common type of hip prostheses implanted comprises a highly polished metallic femoral head which articulates against an ultra high molecular weight polyethylene (UHMWPE) acetabular cup. In the early 1960s Sir John Charnley pioneered the low friction arthroplasty technique, and the introduction of UHMWPE as the bearing surface of the acetabulum has allowed total joint arthroplasty to become the commonplace operation that it is today.

Polyethylene is a semicrystalline polymer of ethylene that is used in orthopaedics because of its superior mechanical and wear properties. In addition, UHMWPE also has a remarkably low frictional coefficient when sliding against metal. However, polyethylene does wear with use. Clinical wear rates (penetration) of explanted failed polyethylene cups have been reported to be in the order of 0.19 mm per year [1, 2]. Radiological studies of normally functioning hips have shown wear rates of approximately half this value [3]. Wear rates are generally higher in younger more active patients and increase with duration after surgery [1, 4]. The release of UHMWPE wear particles from the articulating surfaces of metal on UHMWPE hip prostheses has been shown to elicit a biological response, which ultimately leads to osteolysis, loosening and failure of the prosthesis [5–8]. In normal healthy bone, there is a balance between the activity of the bone forming cells, the osteoblasts, and the bone resorbing cells, the osteoclasts. Poly-

ethylene particles in the size range 0.1–10 μm are phagocytosed by macrophages leading to the release of inflammatory mediators, including cytokines and prostaglandins, which act upon the bone resorbing cells, the osteoclasts, leading to osteolysis [9–11]. Mediators identified as playing a role in bone resorption include, prostaglandin E_2 (PGE_2), cytokines such as tumour necrosis factor-α (TNF-α), interleukin 1 (IL-1), and IL-6, transforming growth factors (TGF-α and TGF-β), colony-stimulating factors (CSF) and enzymes such as collagenase. TNF-α and IL-1 have been shown to be potent stimulators of bone resorption, both in vivo [12] and in vitro [13]. They are often termed osteoclast-activating factors, and IL-1 has also been shown to have an inhibitory effect on osteoblast function and bone collagen synthesis [14]. Monocyte colony-stimulating factor (M-CSF) and granulocyte–monocyte colony-stimulating factor (GM-CSF) have a stimulatory effect on the growth and differentiation of osteoclast precursors, and therefore, are potential regulators of bone resorption [15]. Collagenase has been shown to activate osteoclasts by exposing bone mineral [16]. Conversely, TGF-β inhibits osteoclast formation and high doses of PGE_2 directly inhibit osteoclast activation [16]. There is also evidence to suggest that macrophages are capable of resorbing bone directly by the release of oxide radicals and hydrogen peroxide [17–19].

The volume, size, morphology and concentration of wear particles produced are likely to be dependent on tribological factors such as the material properties, and the loads and motions experienced at the contact surfaces. Wear and the detachment of UHMWPE wear particles can be considered as failure of the polymer material due to cyclic stress fields. Three different wear processes have been identified: (1) wear produced by microscopic counterface asperities; (2) macroscopic polymer asperity wear; and (3) structural failure [20].

Microscopic Counterface Asperity Wear

Microscopic asperities on the femoral counterface produce small scale cyclic stress fields at or near the polymer surface. During sliding of the smooth femoral counterface over the polymer the microscopic asperities repeatedly deform the polymer surface. The polymer surface interacts with many counterface asperities prior to the production of a wear particle, which is produced by fatigue failure [21]. Many micrometre and submicrometre sized particles are predicted to be produced by this process in each articulating cycle of the joint. Rougher femoral counterfaces have larger asperities with larger cyclic stresses, and the wear process may be more abrasive. Consequently fewer interactions are needed to remove the wear particle and the wear rate and volumes are greatly increased.

Macroscopic Polymer Asperity Wear

The surface wear process produced by microscopic counterface asperities assumes that the polymer surface is extremely flat. In reality this is not the case, with typical polymer asperities heights of 1–10 μm being described [20]. The femoral counterface can be considered to be smooth in comparison. Under cyclic loading, the macroscopic polymer asperity is cyclically deformed which produces crack propagation and surface fatigue within 10 μm of the surface. As the dimension of the cyclic stress fields in this process are much larger than in microscopic counterface asperity wear, it is predicted that larger wear particles will be produced by the macroscopic polymer wear process.

Structural Failure

This is a large scale process associated with the overall structural stress field, and is not a surface wear process. However, the failed UHMWPE component can produce large amounts of polymer debris. This structural failure is associated with delamination in replacement knee components and is rarely found in acetabular cups, which have lower levels of contact stress.

There is a clear indication that in order to improve the long-term clinical performance of total artificial joints it is necessary to reduce both the wear of UHMWPE and the number and volume of UHMWPE wear particles generated. In this review, factors affecting the wear of polyethylene such as counterface roughness, sterilisation by gamma irradiation in the presence of air, and the effect these parameters have on the generation of UHMWPE wear particles will be described. In addition, methods of reducing wear and the number of particles generated are also discussed.

Clinical Studies of Wear

There are an increasing number of qualitative studies which describe the role of UHMWPE wear debris in the loosening of total hip prostheses [5, 22, 23]. One study directly related loosening to measured wear volumes in hip prostheses [3]. There have been a number of studies describing the penetration of the femoral head into the acetabular cup. Average penetration rates of 60–100 μm per year have been reported, but the variation can be as great as 10–500 μm [3, 24]. Clinical studies of the Charnley prostheses have revealed penetration rates of 60 μm per year, which corresponds to a maximum wear volume of 20 mm^3 [20]. Average values for larger diameter heads have been described in the range of 10–30 mm^3 per year. If the particles generated have a mean size of less than 1 μm, this wear volume would generate > 10^{10} particles per year, leading to adverse biological reactions and eventual loosening and failure of the prosthesis.

The roughness of the femoral counterface has been shown to be one of the most important determinants of both wear volume and the number of wear particles generated [25, 26]. Clinical studies have shown that if the femoral head remains smooth in vivo polyethylene wear rates are very low [27]. However, in vivo femoral heads can be damaged and roughened by third body particles such as bone cement [24, 28, 29], bone particles [29] and metallic debris from the femoral component [30].

In a recent study, polyethylene wear debris, wear rate of the acetabular cup and femoral head damage were analysed within the same prosthesis for the first time [31]. A series of 18 long-term (implant life 10–19 years) Charnley low friction prostheses, all of which were revised for loosening were collected at revision, along with periprosthetic tissue samples. The surface roughness of the femoral heads and the wear volumes of the acetabular cups were measured. In addition, for the first time, the UHMWPE wear debris was quantitatively isolated from the periprosthetic acetabular tissue for each patient. The retrieved prostheses were split into two groups on the basis of femoral head damage by R_{pm} (height above the mean line), low damage heads ($R_{pm} < 0.2$ μm) and highly damaged heads ($R_{pm} > 0.2$ μm). The prostheses with highly damaged femoral heads had significantly higher volumetric wear rates, higher total penetration, penetration rates, wear volumes and also total number of particles produced over the lifetime of the prosthesis. In addition, significantly more particles were generated per year by the prostheses with highly damaged heads. Importantly, it was shown that there was an association between highly damaged heads and the generation of increased numbers of small particles (< 10 μm), indicating that scratched femoral heads are likely to produce more particles in the biologically active size range.

Laboratory Studies

The influence of counterface roughness on the wear of polyethylene was recognised some time ago. In 1987, a laboratory study reported that a single fine scratch on the counterface, 7 mm deep, which was transverse to the direction of sliding, increased the wear rate of UHMWPE by an order of magnitude [32]. Since then it has been shown that scratches as shallow as 2 mm are capable of increasing the wear rate of UHMWPE by up to 30 times in unidirectional tests, and 70 times in reciprocating tests [33].

A second factor that has been shown to adversely effect the wear of UHMWPE is sterilisation by gamma irradiation in the presence of air or oxygen. Over the past two decades UHMWPE components have been primarily sterilised by gamma irradiation in air, which has been shown to induce time-dependent changes that alter the chemical and mechanical properties of polyethylene [34]. During sterilisation with gamma irradiation free radicals are generated, which are long lived and can cause both chain scission and cross-linking of the UHMWPE. In the presence of oxygen, free radicals initiate a series of long term oxidation reactions that can result in chain scission. The degree of oxidation has been shown to depend upon the dose of irradiation [35], post-irradiation age [35] and environmental conditions [34, 36, 37]. The level of oxidation has been shown to vary with depth [37], peaking at approximately 0.2–2 mm below the surface. Indeed, the presence of a subsurface white band shown to be associated with oxidation has been identified in retrieved polyethylene components [37]. Studies have shown that oxidation of polyethylene causes deterioration of important mechanical properties, such as tensile strength [38], impact strength [34], fatigue strength [34, 39], density [34] and Young's

modulus. Increased crystallinity and reduction in fatigue strength due to oxidation predict higher wear of UHMWPE as the degree of oxidation increases.

In addition, the effect of ageing after gamma irradiation has generated considerable interest, with recent studies showing increased wear rates with increased shelf age [40] and accelerated ageing of components [41]. In vivo, third-body damage to the femoral head and ageing of the polyethylene component may combine to produce accelerated wear of the polymer. In a recent study, Besong et al. [42] studied the combined effects of post-irradiation ageing and counterface roughness on the wear of UHMWPE in vitro.

A controlled laboratory study was carried out, in which the wear of UHMWPE that had been irradiated at a standard sterilisation dose of 2.5 Mrad and aged in air for 3 months, 12 months, 6 years and 10 years, was compared to material that had not been sterilised. Wear rates were determined for counterfaces with three different roughnesses, to represent a newly implanted femoral head ($R_a = 0.01$ μm) and heads that had been damaged by third body wear processes in vivo ($R_a = 0.07$ and 0.1 μm). As the age of the material after irradiation in air increased, the wear rate increased significantly compared to the non-irradiated material. The wear rate was 2.5 times greater at 12 months, three times greater at 6 years and 30 times greater at 10 years. Increasing the counterface roughness dramatically increased the wear rate for all material types. Combining increased counterface roughness and ageing increased the wear rate between five ($R_a = 0.07$ μm) and seven times ($R_a = 0.1$ μm) for the 10-year aged material compared to the non-irradiated material. The combined effect of both ageing the UHMWPE and roughening the counterface produced a 2000-fold increase in wear rate, when comparing the non-irradiated material wearing on the smooth counterface and the 10-year aged material wearing on the roughest counterface.

Ageing of the specimens used in this study took place on the shelf and not in the body and it was clear that all cups do not age or degrade at the same rate after irradiation. This may be due to the dose of irradiation used or the initial processing conditions of the UHMWPE. Clearly some shelf ageing will occur for all implants and in some cases it can be up to 5 years before they are implanted. It is generally thought that the degradation rate in vivo may be less than on the shelf, but this remains to be determined.

In addition to the effect that sterilisation by gamma irradiation in air has on the wear of UHMWPE, Besong et al. [43] also investigated the effect that it has on wear particle production. In this study, the volumetric wear rate, the size distribution and number of particles generated from UHMWPE that had been sterilised by gamma irradiation and aged in air were quantitatively compared to the wear and wear debris generated from UHMWPE that had not been irradiated. The UHMWPE pins were run on a roughened (R_a = 0.07 μm) stainless steel counterface to represent a femoral head that had been slightly damaged in vivo. The lubricant was 25% (v/v) bovine serum, which was collected at the end of each test period for wear debris analysis. The wear debris was analysed by defining particle size and shape using length, area and aspect ratio (length/width). Particle size and mass distributions were also determined along with the total number of particles produced. The number of particles produced per unit volume of wear debris (mm^3) and the wear particle factor (number of particles produced per unit load, per unit sliding distance) were also calculated for the two material types.

As described previously [42], the aged irradiated UHMWPE wore significantly more (six times) than the non-irradiated material. Qualitative analysis of the wear particles by scanning electron microscopy indicated that the particles from the two materials were similar in morphology. Small, regular-shaped granules and larger irregular aggregates were isolated from both materials. The mean aspect ratios of the wear particles were 2.0 and 2.6 for the unsterilised and aged irradiated UHMWPE materials, respectively, indicating that the aged irradiated material produced particles that were more elongated in shape. The mode of the size distributions were in the range 0.1–0.5 μm for both materials. However, 85% of the wear particles generated by the aged irradiated material were in this size range compared to only 65% for the non-irradiated material. This indicates that the size distribution of the particles produced by the aged, irradiated UHMWPE was skewed towards the smaller size range. In addition, the percentage mass of particles in the smallest size range was far higher for the aged irradiated UHMWPE than for the non-irradiated material. These particle size distributions had an even greater effect on the number of particles generated by the two materials, with the aged irradiated material producing 5.5-fold more particles per unit volume (mm^3) of wear than the non-irradiated material. In addition, the number of particles produced per unit load, per unit sliding distance (wear particle factor) was 34 times higher for the aged irradiated UHMWPE compared to the non-irradiated material.

The aged irradiated material produced a lower proportion of particles larger than 1 μm compared to the non-irradiated UHMWPE. This accounted for a higher total number of particles per unit of wear volume, as the size distribution was skewed towards the smaller size range, 0.1–0.5 μm, for the aged irradiated UHMWPE. It has been recognised that non-irradiated UHMWPE retains its toughness [39], and this may allow particles to be drawn and deformed before they are released. The aged irradiated UHMWPE has been shown to have lower fatigue resistance [35, 36, 39, 44] and lower toughness, and this material showed disadvantages in terms of increased volumetric wear, reduced size of wear particles and increased numbers of particles generated. The increased number of smaller particles produced by the aged irradiated UHMWPE suggests that a more severe biological response may be initiated as particles in the 0.1–0.5 μm size range have been shown to elicit an earlier response and increased levels of cytokine production [45]. Brach Del Prever et al. [46] also reported a more adverse biological reaction to irradiated material compared to non-irradiated material.

Recent Advances and Current Clinical Alternatives

We are now in an era in which many different types of polymers and sterilisation methods are being developed and introduced into clinical practice. The main thrust of the research has been to reduce the wear volumes of polyethylene, and hence extend the clinical lifetime of the prosthesis. Recent developments include cross-linking of polyethylene, and alternative approaches to sterilisation. Ethylene oxide sterilisation has been introduced by two implant manufacturers and is not considered to significantly degrade the properties of UHMWPE. However, there have been some concerns about the residuals of the sterilisation process. Sterilisation by irradiation and packaging in inert atmospheres such as nitrogen or argon or under vacuum have also been introduced. This is claimed to provide some benefits of cross-linking without generating oxidative degradation. Recent studies have shown that UHMWPE irradiated and packaged in an inert atmosphere produced lower wear than material that had been irradiated in air [47]. In addition, it has been claimed that UHMWPE sterilised by gamma irradiation with vacuum and inert packaging produces lower wear than ethylene oxide sterilised material [48, 49]. The difference in wear rates between recently irradiated and non-irradiated material has been shown to be dependent on the duration of the test and on femoral head roughness [50]. As the degradation of UHMWPE increases with time after sterilisation, comparison of the different sterilisation methods are of limited clinical value unless they introduce real time or accelerated ageing. Blunn and Bell [51] compared UHMWPE that had been gamma irradiated in air and material that had been irradiated in an inert atmosphere and subsequently stabilised, where both materials had undergone accelerated ageing. The material sterilised by irradiating in an inert atmosphere showed a marked reduction in wear. Recently, Fisher et al. [52] compared the wear of UHMWPE sterilised by gas plasma to the conventional method of gamma irradiation in air, for both non-aged and accelerated aged materials. Untreated UHMWPE was used as a control. Wear rates were studied in simple configuration wear tests using smooth (R_a = 0.01–0.015 μm) stainless steel counterfaces. The effect of the ageing and oxidation processes on the material was studied by Fourier transform infrared technique (FTIR). The results showed that much higher levels of oxidative degradation were present in the material irradiated in air and then aged compared to the material sterilised by gas plasma and aged. The gas plasma sterilised material that had been aged had similar low wear rates to the non-sterilised material, indicating that these treatments did not have a significant effect on the wear properties of the UHMWPE. However, irradiating in air produced a significant increase (50%) in the wear factor of the UHMWPE compared to the non-sterilised material. There was a highly significant three-fold increase in the wear rate of UHMWPE that had been sterilised by gamma irradiation in air and then aged compared to the non-irradiated material, the gas plasma sterilised material and the gas plasma sterilised material that had been aged. The results of the FTIR analysis and the wear data indicate that there was no degradation or increase in wear caused by gas plasma sterilisation and ageing. Previous studies of mechanical properties and fatigue resistance also showed that there was no degradation of the material properties of UHMWPE following gas plasma sterilisation. This study concluded that alternative sterilisation procedures, such as gas plasma, were likely to reduce the wear of the polyethylene component in vivo, which may have considerable benefit in reducing the incidence or delaying the onset of wear debris-induced osteolysis. In addition, it has been predicted that sterilisation of UHMWPE by the gas plasma method will reduce the incidence of delamination in knee replacement components when compared to components that were gamma irradiated in air [53].

Cross-linked UHMWPE has also been introduced into clinical practice in order to reduce wear of the polyethylene component. Cross-linked polyethylene may be more resistant to oxidative degradation following irradiation, and it is now believed that the cross-links provide additional resistance to wear under conditions of a multidirectional frictional force. It has been shown that chemical cross-linking reduces the effect of irradiation on the cross-linked network of UHMWPE. Consequently, wear rates for chemically cross-linked UHMWPE acetabular cups have been shown to be much lower than those of control gamma irradiated cups [54]. In addition, Wroblewski et al. [55] reported extremely low clinical wear rates of cross-linked UHMWPE cups that were coupled with 22-mm ceramic femoral heads. Typical penetration rates of 20 μm per year were cited, which corresponds to a wear volume of 10 mm^3 per year. These rates are very low compared to average clinical penetration rates of 100–200 μm per year with wear rates in the range 30–80 mm^3 per year for metallic femoral heads and polyethylene that has been gamma irradiated in air. Recently, McKellop et al. [56] reported that polyethylene cups cross-linked by increased dosage gamma irradiation have decreased wear rates when worn against smooth femoral counterfaces in a hip simulator. However, it has also been shown that acetylene cross-linked polyethylene wears at a reduced rate in simple configuration wear tests against smooth counterfaces, but when the counterface roughness was increased to represent in vivo femoral head damage, the acetylene cross-linked material was shown to wear significantly more than the non-cross-linked material [57].

In addition to the increased wear resistance of the cross-linked polyethylene cups, the low wear rates reported by Wroblewski et al. [55] may be due to the use of small diameter alumina ceramic femoral heads which are very damage resistant. The surface topography of the femoral counterface has been shown to be one of the most important parameters controlling the wear rate of UHMWPE, and as already discussed, small increases in counterface roughness increase both the wear of UHMWPE and the number of wear particles generated. Clinically, third-body damage to metallic femoral heads can be caused by bone cement particles [24, 28, 58], bone particles [29] and metallic wear debris [30]. In vitro testing has shown that ceramic counterfaces are more resistant to third body damage caused by bone cement than metallic femoral counterfaces [29, 59]. More recently, Minakawa et al. [60] compared third body damage and wear of alumina and zirconia ceramic, and stainless steel, cobalt-chrome and titanium femoral heads in vivo. In addition, the effect of simulated third body damage on the wear of UHMWPE in vitro was determined. The alumina ceramic explanted femoral heads showed the lowest wear determined by surface roughness (R_{pm}), followed by the zirconia ceramic heads. The explanted titanium femoral heads showed greatest wear in all areas measured. The surface roughness (R_{pm}) of the metallic femoral heads was statistically significantly higher than the surface roughness of the ceramic femoral heads. In the laboratory studies, third-body damage was simulated by scratching the counterfaces with a diamond stylus. The simulated scratches were comparable to those found on the explanted femoral heads, as determined by R_p (mean height of the scratch lip). The mean R_p for the simulated scratches was ranked in ascending order: alumina ceramic, zirconia ceramic, cobalt–chrome and stainless steel. The stainless steel counterfaces produced significantly greater wear factors of UHMWPE, threefold greater than the cobalt–chrome counterfaces and fivefold greater than the alumina and zirconia ceramic counterfaces. The alumina and zirconia ceramic counterfaces produced the lowest wear factors of UHMWPE, indicating that the ceramic counterfaces are more resistant to third-body damage than metallic counterfaces. It was also shown that the wear rate of the UHMWPE was dependent on the amount of damage to the counterface (R_p). It is not possible to predict clinical wear rates from simple configuration wear tests, as in vivo many other tribological factors can accelerate wear. However, there are several reports that show that ceramic femoral heads significantly reduce polyethylene wear in hip prostheses clinically [55, 61, 62]. Clearly, alumina and zirconia ceramics are more resistant to third-body damage than metallic alloys and produce less polyethylene wear. It can therefore be predicted that these ceramics have the potential to produce lower long-term clinical wear rates of UHMWPE, thus increasing the implant life of total hip prostheses.

Despite the development and introduction of new polymers into clinical practice, and the introduction of different sterilisation methods, it is necessary to evaluate the tribological performance of these alternative materials in terms of the morphology, size and number of wear particles generated. In addition, it is necessary to determine the biological reactivity of these particles, as a prosthesis that produces decreased wear volumes, but increased numbers of small biologically active wear particles (< 10 μm) may still fail at the same rate as one that produces greater wear volumes but smaller numbers of biologically active particles. The development of a prosthesis that produces both low wear volumes and low numbers of small particles has the potential to significantly increase the implant life of the prosthesis.

These recent advances in prosthesis design, femoral head materials, modified polyethylenes and improved sterilisation methods should provide over 20 years of osteolysis-free life in patients over the age of 65 years. However, for the younger patients

(under 65 years) with life expectancies well beyond 20 years, further improvements in polyethylenes or alternative materials such as metal-on-metal or ceramic-on-ceramic need to be considered. Further research is needed to determine the osteolytic potential of these alternative approaches.

Acknowledgements

The research work cited in this paper that has been carried out at the University of Leeds has been supported by the Arthritis Research Campaign UK, the EC Brite Euram Programme, the DTI CAM1 Programme and the John Charnley Trust.

References

1. Charnley J, Halley DK. Rate of wear in total hip replacement. Clin Orthop 1975;112:170–179.
2. Wroblewski BM, Lynch M, Atkinson JR, Dowson D, Isaac GH. External wear of the polyethylene socket in cemented total hip arthroplasty. J Bone Joint Surg 1987;69B:61–63.
3. Livermore J, Ilstrup D, Morrey B. Effect of femoral head size on wear of the polyethylene acetabular component. J Bone Joint Surg 1990;72A:518–528.
4. Weightman B, Swanson SA, Isaac GH, Wroblewski BM. Polyethylene wear from retrieved acetabular cups. J Bone Joint Surg 1991;73B:806–810.
5. Amstutz HC, Campbell P, Kossovsky N, Clarke IC. Mechanism and clinical significance of wear debris-induced osteolysis. Clin Orthop 1992;276:7–18.
6. Maloney WJ, Jasty M, Rosenberg A, Harris WH. Bone lysis in well-fixed cemented femoral components. J Bone Joint Surg 1990;72B:966–970.
7. Schmalzried TP, Jasty M, Harris WH. Periprosthetic bone loss in total hip arthroplasty. Polyethylene wear debris and the concept of the effective joint space. J Bone Joint Surg 1992;74A:849–863.
8. Schmalzried TP, Kwong LM, Jasty M et al. The mechanism of loosening of cemented acetabular components in total hip arthroplasty. Analysis of specimens retrieved at autopsy. Clin Orthop 1992274:60–78.
9. Green T, Fisher J, Ingham E. Polyethylene particles of a critical size are necessary for the induction of IL-6 by macrophages in vitro. Trans 43rd Orthop Res Soc 1997;22:733.
10. Athanasou NA, Quinn J, Bulstrode CJ. Resorption of bone by inflammatory cells derived from the joint capsule of hip arthroplasties. J Bone Joint Surg 1992;74B:57–62.
11. Murray DW, Rushton N. Mediators of bone resorption around implants. Clin Orthop 1992;281:295–304.
12. Boyce BF, Aufdemorte TB, Garrett IR, Yates AJ, Mundy GR. Effects of interleukin-1 on bone turnover in normal mice. Endocrinology 1989;125:1142–1150.
13. Gowen M, Wood DD, Ihrie EJ, McGuire MK, Russell RG. An interleukin 1 like factor stimulates bone resorption in vitro. Nature 1983;306:378–380.
14. Stashenko P, Dewhirst FE, Rooney ML, Desjardins LA, Heeley JD. Interleukin-1 beta is a potent inhibitor of bone formation in vitro. J Bone Miner Res 1987;2:559–565.
15. Macdonald BR, Mundy GR, Clark S et al. Effects of human recombinant CSF-GM and highly purified CSF-1 on the

formation of multinucleated cells with osteoclast characteristics in long term bone marrow cultures. J Bone Miner Res 1986;1:227–233.

16. Vaes G. Cellular biology and biochemical mechanism of bone resorption. A review of recent developments on the formation, activation and mode of action of osteoclasts. Clin Orthop 1988;231:239–271.

17. Coe MR, Fechner RE, Jeffrey JJ, Balian G, Whitehill R. Characterisation of tissue from the bone-polymethylmethacrylate interface in a rat experimental model. Demonstration of collagen-degrading activity and bone resorbing potential. J Bone Joint Surg 1989;71A:863–874.

18. Horton JE, Raisz LG, Simmons HA, Oppenheim JJ, Mergenhagen SE. Bone resorbing activity in supernatant fluid from cultured peripheral blood leukocytes. Science 1972;177:793–795.

19. Mundy GR, Altman AJ, Gondek MD, Bandelin JG. Direct resorption of bone by human monocytes. Science 1977; 196:1109–1111.

20. Fisher J. Wear of ultra high molecular weight polyethylene in total artificial joints. Curr Orthop 1994;8:164–169.

21. Cooper JR, Dowson D, Fisher J. Macroscopic and microscopic wear mechanisms in ultra-high molecular weight polyethylene. Wear 1993;162:378–384.

22. Lee JM, Salvati EA, Betts F, DiCarlo EF, Doty SB, Bullough PG. Size of metallic and polyethylene debris particles in failed cemented total hip replacements. J Bone Joint Surg 1992;74B:380–384.

23. Shanbhag AS, Jacobs JJ, Glant TT, Gilbert JL, Black J, Galante JO. Composition and morphology of wear debris in failed uncemented total hip replacement. J Bone Joint Surg 1994;76B:60–67.

24. Atkinson JR, Dowson D, Isaac GH, Wroblewski BM. Laboratory wear tests and clinical observations of the penetration of femoral heads into acetabular cups in total replacement hip joints. Wear 1985;104:225–244.

25. Fisher J, Dowson D, Hamdzah H, Lee HL. The effect of sliding velocity on the friction and wear of UHMWPE for use in total artificial joints. Wear 1994;175:219–225.

26. Hailey JL, Ingham E, Stone MH, Wroblewski BM, Fisher J. Ultra-high molecular weight polyethylene wear debris generated in vivo and in laboratory tests; the influence of counterface roughness. Proc Instn Mech Engrs 1996; 210H:3–10.

27. Wroblewski BM, McCullagh PJ, Siney PD. Quality of the surface finish of the head of the femoral component and the wear rate of the socket in long term results of the Charnley low friction arthroplasty. Proc Instn Mech Engrs 1992;206H:181–183.

28. Isaac GH, Atkinson JR, Dowson D, Wroblewski BM. The role of cement in the long term performance and premature failure of Charnley low friction arthroplasties. Eng Med 1986;15:19–22.

29. Caravia L, Dowson D, Fisher J, Jobbins B. The influence of bone and bone cement debris on counterface roughness in sliding wear tests of ultra-high molecular weight polyethylene on stainless steel. Proc Instn Mech Engrs 1990; 204H:65–70.

30. Jasty M, Bragdon CR, Lee K, Hanson A, Harris WH. Surface damage to cobalt chrome femoral head prostheses. J Bone Joint Surg 1994;76B:73–77.

31. Tipper JL, Ingham E, Hailey JL et al. Quantitative comparison of polyethylene wear debris, wear rate and head damage in retrieved hip prostheses. Trans 43rd Orthop Res Soc 1997;22:355.

32. Dowson D, Taheri S, Wallbridge NC. The role of counterface imperfections in the wear of polyethylene. Wear 1987;119:277–293.

33. Fisher J, Firkins PJ, Reeves EA, Hailey JL, Isaac GH. The influence of scratches to metallic counterfaces on the wear of ultra-high molecular weight polyethylene. Proc Instn Mech Engrs 1995;209H:263–264.

34. Rimnac CM, Klein RW, Betts F, Wright TM. Post irradiation ageing of ultra high molecular weight polyethylene. J Bone Joint Surg 1994;76A:1052–1056.

35. Furman B, Li S. The effects of long term shelf life ageing of UHMWPE. Trans 21st Soc Biomaterials, 1995; 114.

36. Trieu HH, Avent RT, Paxson RD. Effects of sterilisation on shelf aged UHMWPE tibial inserts. Trans 21st Soc Biomaterials, 1995; 109.

37. Sun DC, Schmidig G, Stark C, Dumbleton JH. On the origins of subsurface oxidation maximum and its relationship to the performance of UHMWPE implants. Trans 21st Soc Biomaterials, 1995; 362.

38. Pascaud RS, Evans WT, McCullagh PJJ. An investigation into the tensile/compressive properties of UHMWPE as used in TJR's. Trans 21st Soc Biomaterials, 1995; 108.

39. Goldman M, Ranganathan R, Pruitt L, Gronsky R. Characterisation of the structure and fatigue resistance of aged and irradiated UHMWPE. Trans 21st Soc Biomaterials, 1995; 111.

40. Fisher J, Chan KL, Hailey JL, Shaw D, Stone MH. A preliminary study of the effects of ageing following irradiation on the wear of ultra-high molecular weight polyethylene. J Athroplasty 1995;10:689–692.

41. Fisher J, Reeves EA, Isaac GH, Saum KA, Sanford WM. Comparison of the wear of aged and non-aged UHMWPE sterilised with gamma irradiation and gas plasma. Transactions of the 5th World Biomaterials Congress, 1996; 971.

42. Besong AA, Hailey JL, Ingham E, Stone MH, Wroblewski BM, Fisher J. A study of the combined effects of shelf ageing following irradiation in air and counterface roughness on the wear of UHMWPE. Biomed Mater Eng 1997;7:59–65.

43. Besong AA, Tipper JL, Ingham E, Stone MH, Wroblewski BM, Fisher J. Quantitative comparison of wear debris from UHMWPE that has and has not been sterilised by gamma irradiation. J Bone Joint Surg 1998;80B:340–344.

44. Trieu HH, Buchanan DJ, Needham DA et al. Accelerated fatigue wear of gamma-sterilised UHMWPE tibial components. Trans 7th Eur Orthop Res Soc 1997; 106.

45. Green TR, Matthews JB, Fisher J, Ingham E. Cytokine production by macrophages in response to clinically relevant UHMWPE debris of different sizes. Trans 44th Orthop Res Soc 1998;23:374.

46. Brach Del Prever E, Costa L, Galliano P. Ethylene oxide sterilisation of polyethylene cups versus gamma irradiation: different behaviour in vivo. Trans 3rd Eur Fed Orthop Traumatol 1997; 585.

47. Hamilton JV, Schmidt MB, Greer KW. Improved wear of UHMWPE using a vacuum sterilisation process. Trans 42nd Orthop Res Soc 1996;21:20.

48. Schroeder DW, Pozorski KM. Hip simulator testing of isostatically molded UHMWPE: Effect of ETO and gamma irradiation. Trans 42nd Orthop Res Soc 1996;21:478.

49. Sommerich R, Flyn T, Schmidt MB, Zalenski E. The effects of sterilisation on contact area and wear rate of UHMWPE. Trans 42nd Orthop Res Soc1996 21:486.

50. Wang A, Polineni VK, Stark C, Dumbleton JH. Effect of femoral head surface roughening on the wear of unirradiated and gamma irradiated UHMWPE acetabular cups. Trans 42nd Orthop Res Soc 1996;21:473.

51. Blunn GW, Bell CJ. The effect of oxidation on the wear of untreated and stabilised UHMWPE. Trans 42nd Orthop Res Soc 1996;21:482.

52. Fisher J, Reeves EA, Isaac GH, Saum KA, Sanford WM. Comparison of the wear of aged and non-aged ultra high

molecular weight polyethylene sterilised by gamma irradiation and by gas plasma. J Mater Sci: Mater Med 1997; 8:375–378.

53. Reeves EA, Barton DC, FitzPatrick DP, Fisher J. Comparison of gas plasma and gamma irradiation in air sterilisation on the delamination wear of UHMWPE knee replacement components. Trans 44th Orthop Res Soc 1998;23:778.

54. Shen FW, McKellop HA, Salovey R. Irradiation of chemically cross-linked ultrahigh molecular weight polyethylene. J Polymer Sci, Part B Polymer Phys 1996;34:1063–1077.

55. Wroblewski BM, Siney PD, Dowson D, Collins SN. Prospective clinical and joint simulator studies of a new total hip arthroplasty using alumina ceramic heads and cross-linked polyethylene cups. J Bone Joint Surg 1996;78B: 280–285.

56. McKellop H, Shen FW, Salovey R. Extremely low wear of gamma-crosslinked/remelted UHMW polyethylene acetabular cups. Trans 44th Orthop Res Soc 1998;23:98.

57. Marrs H, Barton DC, Ward IM, Doyle C, Fisher J. Comparative wear under three different tribological condi-

tions of acetylene cross-linked ultra high molecular weight polyethylene. Trans 44th Orthop Res Soc 1998;23:100.

58. Isaac GH, Atkinson JR, Dowson D, Kennedy PD, Smith MR. The causes of femoral head roughening in explanted Charnley hip prostheses. Eng Med 1987;16:167–173.

59. Cooper JR, Dowson D, Fisher J, Jobbins B. Ceramic bearing surfaces in total artificial joints: Resistance to third body wear damage from bone cement particles. J Med Eng Tech 1991;15:63–67.

60. Minakawa H, Stone MH, Wroblewski BM, Lancaster JG, Ingham E, Fisher J. Quantification of third body damage and its effect on UHMWPE wear with different types of femoral heads. Trans 43rd Orthop Res Soc 1997;22:788.

61. Schuller HM, Marti RK. Ten year socket wear in 66 hip arthroplasties. Ceramic versus metal heads. Acta Orthop Scand 1990;61:240–243.

62. Oonishi H, Takayama Y, Clarke IC, Jung H. Comparative wear studies of 28 mm ceramic and stainless steel total hip joint over a 2 to 7 year period. J Long-term Med Implant 1992;19:467–476.

11. Metal on Metal Articulation in Total Hip Replacement

P. Roberts and P. Grigoris

An Historical Perspective

The history of metal on metal articulation began at the Middlesex Hospital in London in 1938. Philip Wiles carried out total hip replacements in six patients with Still's disease [1]. The acetabular and femoral components were made of stainless steel and were ground together to ensure an accurate fit. The cup was fixed with two screws and the femoral component was secured by a bolt inserted down the femoral neck, attached to a plate on the lateral aspect of the femur (Fig. 11.1). Unfortunately all the radiographs were lost during the Second World War. Only one patient, with a disintegrated prosthesis, was still alive in 1951. In 1957 Wiles developed another design with better engineering and a more robust method of fixation. He performed eight operations, but the results were disappointing because of bone resorption and prosthetic loosening.

A similar stainless steel implant was used by Kenneth Coutts in Boston, USA [2]. He implanted one prosthesis that was revised 6 years postoperatively. In 1951 Edward Haboush at the Hospital for Joint Diseases in New York inserted a Vitallium total hip replacement with accurately matched articulating surfaces. Both components were fixed with Cranioplast®, a type of polymethylmethacrylate cement, which at the time was used for the repair of skull defects. The joint dislocated in the early postoperative period because of a vertically positioned acetabular component and the construct never actually functioned.

In the early 1950s Kenneth McKee, who had worked with Wiles as his Senior Registrar, implanted three metal on metal hip replacements based on his hip arthrodesis screw [3, 4]. Two were made from stainless steel and these became loose within 1 year. The

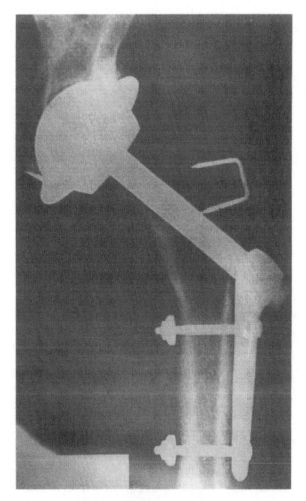

Fig. 11.1. The Wiles total hip replacement.

third prosthesis was fixed with cobalt–chrome screws and survived for three years. McKee was instrumental in promoting the idea of total hip replacement during the 1950s, when Charnley was rather pessimistic, advocating central dislocation of the hip to achieve arthrodesis for degenerative osteoarthritis.

In 1953 McKee visited the United States and played golf with Thompson. After his return to Norwich, he matched his cobalt–chrome clover-leaf socket to a modified Thompson stem with a 1¼ inch diameter head. Between 1956 and 1960 McKee implanted 26 of these press fit hips. Over a period of 7 years, 15 were reported to be satisfactory and 10 failed and were revised [5].

In 1960 McKee made changes to the design of the acetabular component so that it could be used with bone cement. The eventual design was a hemispherical cup with a lip and with small studs on the outer surface. This was paired with a standard Thompson prosthesis with a head diameter of 1 and 5/8 inches (Fig. 11.2). The wide-neck geometry of the femoral component and the full hemispherical acetabular component made anterior impingement a common occurrence. In a series of one hundred patients undergoing total hip replacement between 1961 and 1964 using this prosthesis, there were thirty

revisions, of which McKee attributed sixteen to prosthetic impingement [5].

In 1965 the neck of the femoral component was recessed in an attempt to reduce impingement. This was the contribution of Watson-Farrar (Fig. 11.3). At this time the components were sold as matched pairs, lapped together for an accurate fit. In 1966 smaller sized components were introduced in an attempt to improve the bony support of the acetabular component [6].

In 1956 Scales and Wilson worked on the development of a metal on metal articulation at the Royal National Orthopaedic Hospital, Stanmore [1, 7]. The first components were implanted in 1963. The acetabular component was initially made in two parts and was designed for use without cement. In 1966 a one-piece cup for cemented use was introduced. A concave, horse-shoe bearing surface on the cup was adopted. The relieved portion was intended to permit ingress of lubrication to the inner bearing surfaces and provide egress for wear debris. The articulating surfaces were ground and then lapped together, resulting in equatorial bearing. This component was associated with a high incidence of early prosthetic loosening and seizure of some of the components [8].

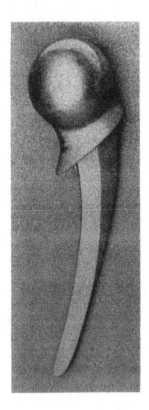

Fig. 11.2. Thompson prosthesis as used initially by McKee.

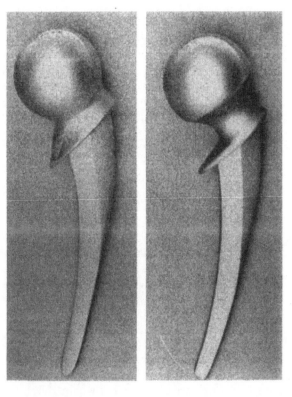

Fig. 11.3. Evolution of the Thompson prosthesis with reduction in the neck diameter.

In 1968 the acetabular component was modified: the clearance between the head and socket was increased and the pole of the socket was relieved to provide an annular bearing area (Fig. 11.4). The engineering practice of finishing the bearing surfaces was also dramatically improved [9, 10]. In 1980 Dobbs retrospectively reviewed the entire series from Stanmore, comprising 173 metal on metal implants of various developmental designs [11]. The prosthetic survival at 11 years was 53%. Loosening occurred mostly on the acetabular side. With comparable follow-up, the overall incidence of revision using the horse-shoe equatorial bearing was 58%, compared to 15% using the 1968 polar bearing design.

Peter Ring at Redhill, Surrey, introduced a metal on metal articulation in 1964 [12, 13]. The acetabular component had a long threaded stem that was used to gain fixation in the iliopubic bar of the pelvis.

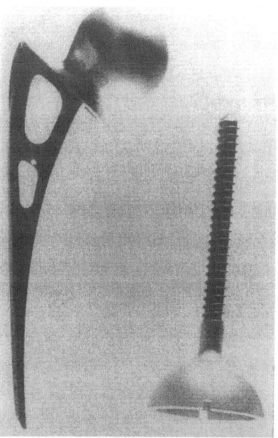

Fig. 11.5. Original version of the Ring total hip replacement (Mark 1).

This was used in conjunction with a standard Austin–Moore prosthesis with a 40 mm head (Fig. 11.5). Both components were manufactured from cobalt–chrome alloy and were inserted without cement. The components were lapped together resulting in equatorial bearing. One hundred and eighty five of these implants were inserted. After 11 to 14 years follow-up there were reported to be 38% poor results, including revisions [14].

In 1967 the acetabular component was modified to a conical shape, with a thicker, tapered stem. The neck shaft angle of the femoral component was increased to 150° in an attempt to lower the incidence of femoral component loosening. Equatorial bearing was also abandoned in favour of polar bearing, with a clearance of approximately 500 μm. The outcome of this series was improved, with 80% prosthetic survival at 17 years [15]. However, the reduced offset of the stem frequently caused a poor gait and a valgus deformity of the knee often developed. In 1971 the definitive femoral component was introduced: this had a neck shaft angle of 135° (Fig. 11.6).

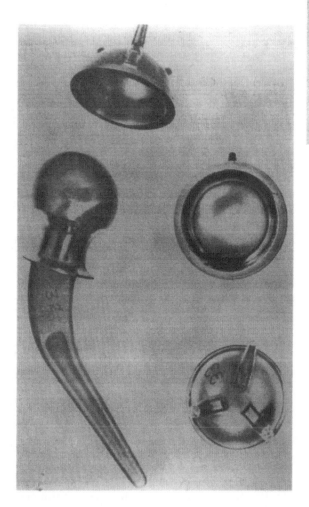

Fig. 11.4. Final version of the Stanmore metal on metal total hip replacement.

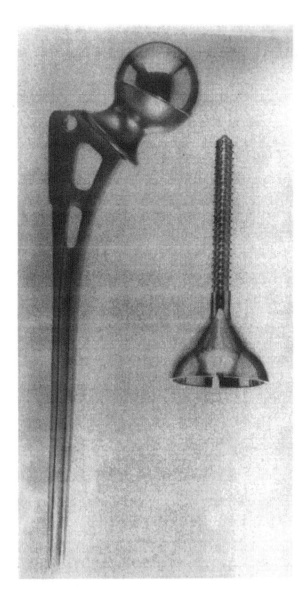

Fig. 11.6. Definitive Ring total hip replacement (Mark IV).

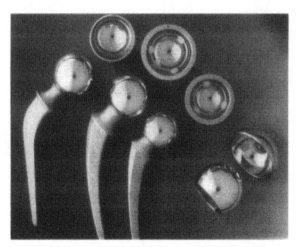

Fig. 11.7. The range of Huggler and Muller metal on metal total hip replacements. From left to right: (i) Huggler prosthesis 42-mm head; (ii) Muller prosthesis 42-mm head; (iii) Muller prosthesis 37-mm head; (iv) Muller resurfacing prosthesis.

In 1965, Arnold Huggler and Maurice Muller, in conjunction with Sulzer Brothers, developed metal on metal hip prostheses for use with bone cement. The Huggler design was based on a Charnley type stem, whilst Muller used a modified McKee stem (Fig. 11.7). Both prostheses were made from cast cobalt–chrome alloy, with highly polished articulating surfaces. The inner side of the cup also had three polyacetal sliding bearings, designed to enhance lubrication. The articulation was available in diameters of 37 mm and 42 mm. From the outset polar bearing was achieved with a clearance of between 0.12 mm and 0.5 mm [16, 17].

In 1967 Muller designed a metal on metal resur-

facing prosthesis for use in young patients. Muller implanted 35 stemmed and 18 surface replacements, but despite early excellent results he abandoned the use of the all metal articulation in favour of a metal on polyethylene articulation in 1968. Six of these all metal articulations were revised after functioning for up to 25 years [18, 19].

In a study from Uppsala, Sweden, Almby and Hierton reported on 107 consecutive Muller-McKee arthroplasties performed between 1967 and 1970 [20]. After a minimum 10-year follow up there were 29 revisions for aseptic loosening, including four for stem fracture.

In 1959, KM Sivash in Moscow began to implant an all metal prosthesis in which the femoral head was "captured" in the acetabular component to prevent dislocation (Fig. 11.8). The implant was initially manufactured from stainless steel, but later cobalt–chrome alloy was used [21]. In 1969 Sivash reported on 200 hips with a maximum follow-up of 9 years. There were 13 stem fractures and seven infections. The prosthesis never gained wide popularity outside the Soviet Union, but it was used by several surgeons in the south-eastern part of the United States. It later led to the development of the S-ROM stem.

In France, Merle D'Aubigné modified the McKee prosthesis and introduced its use in 1965 [22]. The femoral stem was a Moore type without a fenestration. There was only one head size with a diameter of 41 mm. A study of 113 of these prostheses, inserted at the Hôpital Cochin, Paris, with an average follow-up of nine years, reported a 30% aseptic loosening rate, including revisions.

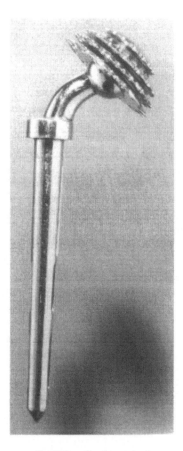

Fig. 11.8. Sivash prosthesis.

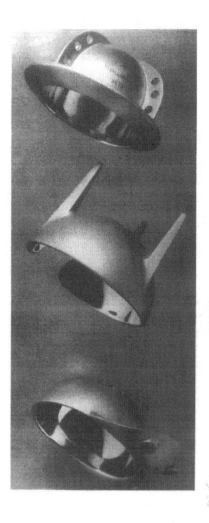

Fig. 11.9. Vitallium hemiarthroplasties. From above: (i) McBride; (ii) Urist; (iii) Gaenslen.

In the United States in the 1950s and 1960s, the McBride, Gaenslen and Urist cups were used in several centres as acetabular hemiarthroplasties (Fig. 11.9). The Thompson, Austin–Moore and Leinbach femoral prostheses were also in common use for the treatment of hip fractures and for hip arthritis. In the 1960s these acetabular and femoral components were used in different combinations to carry out total joint replacements [23–28]. At this time the components were variably matched by the manufacturers. Initially they were lapped together, but by the end of the 1960s a polar bearing design with apical and equatorial relief was adopted. The published reports from the United States noted good functional results with a variable reoperation rate. The French experience with a Urist cup and an unmatched Austin-Moore femoral component was less good: up to 50% failure within 3 years was reported [29].

Problems with the Early Metal on Metal Articulations

The first generation of metal on metal total hip replacements was associated with a high rate of early loosening. Various factors were responsible:

Materials

The Wiles' hip, the early versions of the McKee and the early versions of the Sivash were manufactured from stainless steel. This material was associated with very high wear of the bearing surfaces, high friction and corrosion. In contrast, cobalt–chrome molybdenum alloys have the necessary metallurgical characteristics to be used in bearing couples. Since the late 1950s all metal on metal bearings have been manufactured from such alloys.

Bearing Design

A common feature of the early metal on metal total hip replacements used in the United Kingdom before 1968 was the small clearance (radial mismatch) between the head and the socket. The initial Stanmore prostheses were ground and lapped together to ensure equatorial bearing. In 1965 the McKee prostheses were sold as matched pairs and were said to be "lapped". The early Ring prostheses were also said to have been lapped together, resulting in equatorial bearing of the components. These designs were commonly associated with excessive wear of the articulating surfaces and early loosening of the components.

By 1967 the problems associated with equatorial bearing were recognised. Ring introduced a diametric mismatch of approximately 0.5 mm between the femoral and acetabular components to ensure "polar" bearing [30]. Likewise, the geometry of the McKee and the Stanmore designs was changed to ensure polar rather than equatorial bearing. These observations were confirmed in 1971, when Walker and Gold reported that equatorial bearing of a metal on metal articulation generated a frictional torque many times greater than that when polar bearing occurred [31]. In general, the good results that have been published from metal on metal bearings have been from those prostheses with polar bearing.

In 1971 Postel at the Hôpital Cochin in Paris designed a metal on metal hip replacement using a "low friction band" (*bandes du glissement*). The articular surface of the socket had raised concentric bands with the intention of avoiding the potential point contact of polar bearing prostheses and to act as lubrication channels. This design modification led to disappointing results (39% failure at $5\frac{1}{2}$ years), due to excessive wear of the acetabular component [32].

The Decline of Metal on Metal Bearings

By the early 1970s excellent early results of the Charnley low friction arthroplasty were being reported and the use of metal on metal articulations was in decline. Every year hundreds of surgeons visited Wrightington Hospital and were taught by Charnley the theoretical basis and the surgical technique of his operation. This included the famous demonstration of frictional torque using a pendulum comparator, in which the McKee metal on metal prosthesis ground rapidly to a halt whilst a Charnley prosthesis continued to swing.

Until the early 1970s only selected surgeons were permitted to implant the Charnley prosthesis. Charnley stressed the importance of cup medialisation to reduce the joint reaction force, bony containment of the cup and correct alignment of the femoral stem. In contrast, McKee never restricted the use of his prosthesis. His surgical technique frequently resulted in unsupported cups, particularly when only one size was available, and neck impingement. Together with the problems of irregular geometry, poor surface finish and the equatorial bearing of the early designs, this resulted in higher early failure rates compared to the Charnley prosthesis.

McKee ceased using his metal on metal hip on his retirement in 1972. Ring abandoned his metal on metal articulation in favour of a metal on polythene bearing in 1979. By that time metal on metal bearings had also largely been abandoned in the United States and Europe.

Whilst the tribological behaviour of the first generation of metal on metal hip replacements undoubtedly contributed to the early loosening of these components, there were other factors, unrelated to the bearing, which contributed to the relatively poor results achieved with the McKee prosthesis compared to Charnley's low friction arthroplasty. The McKee stem was curved with narrow medial and lateral borders and multiple sharp corners. In addition, the broad neck was prone to impingement on the edge of the acetabular component. In comparison, the Charnley stem was straight, with a gentle taper. It had broad medial and lateral surfaces and smooth contours, characteristics which are now known to be desirable for the femoral component.

Renaissance of Metal on Metal Bearings

By the early 1980s it was apparent that many metal on metal hip replacements of the post-1968 era were functioning well, without the radiographic changes of periprosthetic osteolysis that we now attribute to the effects of submicron polyethylene wear debris.

In 1985 Semlitsch, Streicher and Weber [16] analysed explants of 6 Huggler and 11 Muller metal on metal prostheses which had been in use for up to 20 years. With the exception of one Huggler prosthesis with a clearance of 0.5 mm, all the other explants had a clearance of between 0.12 and 0.2 mm. Excluding the Huggler prosthesis with its excessive clearance, the average maximal linear wear rate was of the order of 2.5 to 5 μm per year for a femoral component with a 42 mm diameter head.

This is approximately 40 times less than the average linear wear rate found in explants of Muller prostheses with a cobalt–chrome alloy on polyethylene articulation, with a 32 mm diameter head.

Schmidt, Weber and Schon carried out a retrieval analysis of 30 McKee-Farrar and 24 Muller all metal total hip replacements [33]. Using a co-ordinate measuring machine they found that the total average linear wear rate of the head and socket together was 12 μm for the McKee Farrar prosthesis and 4 μm for the Muller. The average clearance was 120 ± 40 μm for the McKee-Farrar prostheses and 210 ± 50 μm for the Muller prostheses. Similarly, McKellop et al. [34] reported a mean linear wear rate of 6 μm per year for 21 metal on metal hip replacements of various designs (McKee–Farrar, Muller, Ring and Huggler), which had been implanted for between 1 and 25 years.

Based on the excellent wear results of the retrieved Huggler and Muller prostheses, Bernard Weber, in collaboration with Sulzer Brothers, began the development of a modern all metal hip replacement using the high carbon containing cobalt–chrome wrought forged alloy, Protasul-21WF. In comparison with the original cast cobalt–chrome alloy Protasul-1, Protasul-21WF had smaller carbides with a more homogenous distribution. This offered the potential for the reduction in surface roughness, whilst maintaining high wear resistance. This work led to the development of the Metasul™ bearing, which was first implanted by Weber in 1988 [35]. Since then 85 000 total hip replacements using the Metasul™ bearing have been implanted world-wide.

Several other systems using metal on metal articulations have been introduced: Johnson & Johnson, Stratec, Endo Plus, Biomet, Mathys and Wright Medical have developed total hip replacements. Resurfacing prostheses using metal on metal bearings have been developed in Germany by Wagner (using the Metasul™ bearing) [36] in the United Kingdom by Corin [37] and Midlands Medical Technology, and in the United States by Amstutz, in collaboration with Wright Medical [38, 39].

Contemporary Issues

Metallurgy

The optimal metallurgy for metal on metal bearings is controversial. The major issues are:

1. the carbon content of the cobalt–chrome molybdenum alloy;
2. wrought or cast alloys;
3. the importance of post-casting heat treatments.

High Carbon Versus Low Carbon Cobalt–Chrome Molybdenum Alloys

High carbon containing alloys have approximately 0.2% carbon content. During the manufacturing process the carbon is converted to carbides of chromium and molybdenum. This leads to a biphasic material, in which the carbides, that have ceramic like properties, are distributed throughout the metal matrix. The size and the distribution of the metallic carbides is dependent on the manufacturing process.

Surface carbides have a high hardness and confer resistance to adhesive wear. The metallic matrix in comparison, is relatively soft but is fracture resistant and confers resistance to abrasive wear. The carbide content of low carbon alloys is significantly reduced compared to the carbide content of high carbon alloys. In pin on disc tests, low carbon containing alloys (less than 0.08%) had reduced surface hardness and showed wear rates up to 18 times higher than high carbon containing alloys (greater than 0.2%) [33]. However, in a hip simulator study, Farrar et al. [40] demonstrated no significant difference in total wear rates of acetabular and femoral components when manufactured from low or high carbon containing alloys.

Wrought Versus Cast Alloy

The process of wrought forging results in smaller, more evenly distributed carbide particles within the metal matrix compared to cast alloys. In theory, this leads to increased surface hardness, increased wear resistance and decreased surface roughness after polishing. These are all characteristics desirable of a metal on metal bearing. However, on pin and disc tests there was no significant difference in wear between high carbon containing cast and wrought forged alloys [33].

The Role of Post-casting Heat Treatments

The draft European standard prEN12563.1997 recommends that cast cobalt–chrome molybdenum alloys used for prosthesis manufacture undergo post-casting heat treatments, to improve ductility and to reduce porosity. Hot isostatic pressing and/or solution heat treatments are generally used for this purpose. However, such post-casting heat treatments alter the metallurgical structure of the alloy: solution annealed cobalt–chrome alloy has a substantially lower total volume percent carbide phase, different carbide phases and higher dissolved carbon in the matrix than as-cast cobalt–chrome alloys. These differences result in different hardness gradients in the microstructure. They may also affect the initial surface roughness. These changes in the microstructure and surface characteristics may potentially affect the wear behaviour of the bearing.

Nelson and Dyson [41] have studied the wear characteristics of the Cormet 2000 resurfacing prosthesis, using a Stanmore Mark III hip simulator and a 3-D co-ordinate measuring machine. They found that the cumulative linear wear of a 48-mm diameter bearing, with a 300-μm diametrical mismatch, was similar for a prosthesis manufactured from cast alloy that did not undergo post-casting heat treatment when compared to a prosthesis manufactured from alloy which had undergone post-casting solution heat treatment and hot isostatic pressing. This suggests, that for this prosthesis at least, the metallurgical changes brought about by post-casting annealing do not influence the wear characteristics of the bearing surface. Similar findings have been reported by Bobyn et al. [42].

The Importance of Clearance

An adequate clearance (radial mismatch) is a prerequisite for the long term function of a metal on metal bearing. The rapid failure of many of the early designs occurred because the articulation had inadequate clearance, resulting in equatorial bearing, with associated high wear and friction. By the end of the 1960s the importance of clearance had been recognised and the designs of this era were manufactured with larger clearances to achieve polar bearing.

Theoretical Considerations

The optimal clearance requires a compromise between maximising contact area between the bearing surfaces, whilst avoiding the risk of equatorial bearing. The smaller the clearance (i.e. the smaller the radial mismatch), the greater is the contact area over which the load can be distributed. This should result in lower wear. However, when the clearance between the ball and socket becomes very low, other factors come into play which could result in equatorial bearing :

1. The rim of the socket deforms under load. The magnitude of this deformation can be of the order of 20 μm.
2. Manufacturing tolerances can lead to up to 3 μm of out-of-roundness of the femoral and acetabular components.
3. The presence of large surface asperities (carbides) will reduce the nominal clearance until the asperities are worn away.

In the worst case scenario, if all these factors came into play, equatorial bearing could result if the clearance of a bearing with a 28-mm diameter head was below approximately 50 μm. The minimal clearance for larger components should be greater, because larger acetabular components have more rim deformation under load when compared with smaller acetabular components with the same wall thickness.

Hip Simulator and Retrieval Studies

Using a MMED hip simulator, Farrar et al. analysed the effects of diametrical clearance on wear using a 28-mm head [40]. They found that total wear was minimised when the diametrical clearance ranged between 33 and 150 μm. Outside this range wear increased dramatically.

Retrieval studies of metal on metal bearings have also demonstrated accelerated wear in articulations with excessive clearance. Semlitsch et al. analysed a Huggler prosthesis with a clearance of 500 μm [16]. This prosthesis had a wear rate several times higher than other retrieved Huggler prostheses with clearances between 120 and 200 μm. Likewise, McKellop et al. found that a retrieved McKee–Farrar prosthesis with a clearance of 1748 μm had extreme wear when compared to retrieved McKee–Farrar prostheses with clearances of less than 386 μm [43].

Lubrication

In the non-diseased human hip joint, there is no contact between the articulating surfaces because fluid film lubrication occurs by various mechanisms (boundary lubrication by glycoproteins attaching themselves to the articular surfaces is also important at low loads). True fluid film lubrication does not occur in artificial hip joints, however, some form of lubrication is essential to reduce wear and friction.

Charnley delighted in demonstrating to visiting surgeons how a metal on metal McKee–Farrar prosthesis rapidly ground to a halt on his pendulum comparator, whilst his metal on polyethylene articulation continued to swing. However, it is probable that these tests were run without any lubrication, which is now known to particularly adversely affect metal on metal bearings. Streicher et al. demonstrated in hip simulator tests, that the frictional torque of a metal on metal bearing was halved when lubricated with bovine serum, compared to when run dry [44].

At present the rheology of the lubricating fluid of an implanted metal on metal articulation cannot be influenced. However, certain design features of the metal on metal articulation do influence lubrication.

Clearance

The thickness of the fluid film can be increased by increasing the apparent contact area between the articular surfaces (this reduces the contact pressure) and by reducing the angle of convergence of the contact surfaces. Both these conditions occur when the diametrical mismatch between the components (clearance) is low. However, for the reasons documented above, the clearance of a metal on metal articulation using a 28-mm head should not be reduced below 30 to 50 μm, because equatorial bearing may occur.

Surface Roughness

Micro-topography is critical in maintaining fluid films, particularly if the local conditions result in thin fluid films. If the combined surface roughness of the articulating surfaces is comparable to that of the fluid film thickness, then asperity contact occurs, leading to increased friction and wear. In general, the smoother the surface finish the better the lubrication potential. In theory, if the surfaces were too smooth, then adhesion could occur, but this is most unlikely in contemporary metal on metal articulations, where the surface roughness is of the order of Ra 0.02 to Ra 0.05.

In wrought forged cobalt–chrome molybdenum alloys, the surface carbides are smaller and are more homogeneously distributed when compared to cast alloys of the same chemical composition. Such wrought forged alloys can be polished to a better surface finish than cast alloys. The process of wrought forging may therefore confer enhanced lubrication properties to metal on metal articulations.

Chemical Properties of the Alloy

Metalloprotein compounds have been identified on the articular surfaces of retrieved metal on metal implants. It is possible that such compounds may play some role in allowing boundary lubrication to occur. Unsworth et al. have suggested that it is probable that mixed lubrication mechanisms (i.e. fluid film and boundary) operate in metal on metal articulations [45, 46]. If boundary lubrication does play a significant role, then the chemical properties of the articulating surfaces (in contrast to the physical properties) may become relevant.

Friction

Sir John Charnley promoted his prosthesis as a low frictional torque arthroplasty based on a stainless steel on polyethylene articulation and a small head diameter. He used his pendulum comparator to demonstrate the improved frictional torque characteristics of his bearing compared to the McKee–Farrar metal on metal bearing.

Frictional torque is however dependent on many factors, not least lubrication, clearance and surface finish. More recent analyses of the frictional torque of modern metal on metal articulations have not confirmed the results demonstrated by Charnley's pendulum comparator. Streicher et al. tested various articulations in a Buchs type pendulum apparatus [47]. The parameter assessed was the maximum number of cycles until the pendulum came to rest after its release, without momentum, from an angle of 25° with a load of 800 N. A mixture of Ringer's solution and 30% calf serum was used as a lubricant. A Metasul™ bearing with a head diameter of 37 mm had a 70–100% higher frictional torque than a metal on polyethylene bearing with a head diameter of 32 mm. However, if the head diameter of the metal on metal articulation was reduced to 28 mm, the frictional torque was the same as that of metal on polyethylene and ceramic on polyethylene articulations with a head diameter of 32 mm.

The same authors measured the frictional torque of the same articulations on a Stanmore Mark III hip simulator. Using a 28-mm head, the frictional torque of an all metal articulation was initially of the order of 3 Nm, but after 0.5 million cycles the frictional torque dropped to approximately 1.2–1.5 Nm, and then remained steady. This frictional torque is similar to that measured for a metal on polyethylene articulation.

Nelson and Dyson measured the frictional torque of a Cormet 2000 resurfacing prosthesis with a 48 mm diameter head and a diametrical mismatch of 291 μm [41]. The frictional torque was 6 Nm. If the diametrical mismatch was reduced to 81 μm, the frictional torque rose to 18 Nm. This is still much lower than the static torque required to remove a well-cemented cup from a cadaveric acetabulum: This has been documented by Andersson et al. to be of the order of 100 Nm [48].

The importance of clearance on frictional torque was demonstrated by Walker and Gold [31]. If the clearance is sufficient to allow polar contact, then frictional torque is at a minimum. However, if contact occurs beyond 60° from the pole, frictional torque increases, until at equatorial contact the frictional torque is theoretically infinite.

Wear

Modern metal on metal bearings are characterised by very low wear rates: up to 80 times less than that seen with metal on polyethylene bearings, and similar to that seen in ceramic on ceramic bearings.

Hip Simulator Studies

Rieker et al assessed the wear characteristics of a Metasul™ bearing using a 28-mm head on a Stanmore Mark III hip simulator [49]. The wear was evaluated using a three-dimensional co-ordinate measuring machine, with a spatial resolution of less than 1 μm in the area of measurement. When the clearance between the components was optimal (approximately 100 μm), the total wear after one million cycles approached 25 μm. After this initial "running in period", the total wear rate stabilised between 4 and 10 μm per million cycles.

Nelson and Dyson have measured the wear rate of a Cormet 2000 resurfacing prosthesis with a 48mm diameter head [41]. A Stanmore Mark III hip simulator was used and the linear wear was measured using a co-ordinate measuring machine. They found that following the initial "bedding in period" there was approximately 4 μm per million cycles of wear of the acetabular component, with minimal wear of the femoral component.

Retrieval Analysis

Several authors have studied the wear behaviour of explanted metal on metal bearings. McKellop et al. analysed 21 metal on metal hip replacements of various designs, with up to 25 years use in vivo [34]. The long-term annual linear wear rate was approximately 6 μm. Sieber et al. analysed 118 retrieved specimens of the head or cup of Metasul™ bearings [50]. They found total wear rates of approximately 25 μm for the whole articulation in the first year. This subsequently stabilised to approximately 5 μm per year after the third year.

These results are very similar to the wear rates observed on hip simulator studies on Metasul™ bearings with 28-mm heads. This compares with the linear wear rate of approximately 200 μm per year seen in metal on polyethylene articulations and 100 μm per year seen in ceramic on polyethylene articulations. In Sieber's study the volumetric wear of the Metasul™ bearing was 60-fold less than that seen in metal on polyethylene articulations.

Pattern of Wear

McKellop et al. have analysed the pattern of wear on retrieved metal on metal hip replacements of various designs [34]. Using light and scanning electron microscopy, they found that early wear was largely due to third-body abrasion, possibly from particles generated while scratches from the original polishing were being eradicated and/or from dislodged surface carbides. The main contact zones were eventually worn smoother than the original surfaces, indicating a self-healing/self-polishing phenomenon of the articular surfaces. This self-healing property is a consequence of the high ductility of the cobalt–chrome molybdenum alloy. The self-polishing process, by improving the surface finish over time, results in a reduction of the wear rate.

Walker and Gold documented evidence of equatorial wear on the heads of 10 retrieved McKee–Farrar prostheses [31]. They postulated that, although there was a nominal diametric mismatch between the ball and socket, this was inadequate to permit polar bearing, possibly because of inadequate manufacturing tolerances. Equatorial bearing therefore resulted. This would significantly increase the frictional torque, which could have contributed to the loosening of the prostheses. In contrast, McKellop et al. demonstrated that the superomedial part of the femoral head was the predominant area of wear when there was adequate clearance between the articulating surfaces [34].

Rieker et al. confirmed that scratching due to third body abrasion was the predominant form of wear in retrievals of Metasul™ bearings [49]. They also observed the self-healing effect, in which relatively large scratches (approximately 5 μm in depth and width) were converted to much shallower and narrower scratches by self-polishing of the articular surface. In about 10% of their retrieved specimens they also found evidence of micro-pitting in the weight-bearing area of the femoral head. By scanning electron microscopy and laser profilometry, they demonstrated that these micro-pits were approximately 0.3 to 0.5 μm in depth. It is probable that these micro-pits were a consequence of adhesive or fatigue wear. This adhesive wear did not significantly affect the overall wear rate of the bearings: there was no significant difference in the overall wear rate in bearings in which adhesive or fatigue wear was demonstrated, when compared with bearings in which only abrasive wear was noted.

Wear Particle-induced Osteolysis

Periprosthetic osteolysis has not been a feature of the long-term radiographic analysis of modern metal on metal hip replacements [35]. When revision surgery has been carried out there has been no evidence of the black staining of the periprosthetic tissues commonly associated with metallosis. Whilst the volumetric wear rate of metal on metal articulations is between 60 and 300 times less than that of metal on polyethylene articulations, there is, inevitably, some wear of the articular surfaces.

Doorn et al have estimated the production of wear particles from metal on metal and metal on polyethylene bearings, based on a mean diameter of 0.08 μm for metal particles and 0.5 μm for polyethylene particles [51]. This estimate of particle size is based on various reports in the literature [52]. Using in vitro and in vivo derived wear rates, a metal on metal bearing would produce 1.9×10^{13} particles per year, compared to 1.5×10^{12} polyethylene particles from a metal on polyethylene bearing.

Despite the production of a large number of metal particles, granuloma formation is rarely seen in the periprosthetic tissues around a metal on metal articulation. This may be because the predominant size of the metal particles produced from a metal on metal bearing is too small to activate macrophages. Green, Fisher and Ingham have demonstrated that maximum macrophage activation for the production of interleukin-6 occurs with polyethylene particles in the phagocytosable size range of 0.5 to 10 μm [53]. If this size-specific effect of macrophage stimulation applies to metal particles, then significant cytokine production would not be anticipated around metal on metal bearings, despite the large number of particles produced.

Carcinogenesis

The potential carcinogenic and toxic effects of released metal particles and ions were concerns raised early in the development of total hip replacement. Early studies reported a high incidence of tumours in rats after they had been injected with massive doses of wear particles from Co–Cr prostheses [54]. However similar results have not been reproduced in more recent animal studies [55–57]. It is of relevance that polyethylene and polymethylmethacrylate (PMMA) particles can also cause cancer in rats. Nevertheless, concerns remain about the potential effect of metal wear and/or corrosion products, especially in the long term. If the latency period for tumour induction is approximately 20 years, prolonged exposure to metal may be a problem in young patients.

In 1988 Gillespie et al reported an increased risk for tumours of the lymphatic and haemopoietic system in patients who had undergone metal on metal and metal-on-polyethylene hip replacements [58]. Similar findings were reported by Visuri, who analysed a patient population with McKee–Farrar arthroplasties [59, 60]. In contrast, three other epidemiological studies did not establish any association between metal-on-polyethylene joint replacements and an increased incidence of cancer during the first 10 postoperative years [61–63].

Case et al. reported dissemination of metal debris from implants in lymph nodes, liver, spleen and bone marrow [64, 65]. There is also some evidence suggesting increased metal concentrations in serum and urine in patients with metal on metal articulations compared with patients who had metal-on-polyethylene implants [66, 67]. The clinical significance of these findings is unknown. A possible slight increased risk of haemopoietic cancers in young patients undergoing metal on metal hip replacements must be weighed against the potential benefits of less periprosthetic osteolysis and lower revision rates.

Summary

Metal on metal bearings in total hip replacement surgery have had a chequered history. The early designs were associated with high rates of wear and early prosthetic loosening compared to prostheses using metal on polyethylene bearings. However, when the importance of adequate clearance between the articulating surfaces was recognised and surface finish was improved, excellent long-term results were achieved.

Contemporary metal on metal bearings have very low wear rates of the articulating surfaces, thus minimising the risk of wear debris induced periprosthetic osteolysis. There is therefore the potential for long-term stable fixation to the skeleton. When used as a surface replacement, metal on metal bearings offer both immediate and long term conservation of bone stock.

Questions remain, particularly relating to the optimal metallurgical characteristics of the bearing and the potential long-term toxic effects of metal particles and ions. It would therefore seem appropriate to limit the use of such bearings, at least in the short term, to biologically young, active patients in whom metal on polyethylene bearings perform poorly. Comprehensive long-term clinical studies will be required to assess the performance of the bearing couple and to monitor complications and failures. Investigation of metal ion concentrations in the body fluids of patients with metal on metal bearings will also be necessary.

The resurgence of interest in metal on metal bearings is likely to continue because of the inherent problem of the production of biologically active wear particles from metal on polyethylene articulations. To date there are no published studies of the medium to long-term results of hip replacements using metal on metal bearings. It will be another 10 years before the performance of this bearing can be compared meaningfully with conventional metal on plastic articulations. Until such data are available, metal on metal bearings should continue to be regarded as experimental.

References

1. Scales JT. Arthroplasty of the hip using foreign materials: a history. Symposium on lubrication and wear in living and artificial human joints. London Inst Mech Eng 1967; 63–84.
2. Walker PS. Historical development of artificial joints in human joints and their artificial replacements. Springfield, IL: Thomas, 1977; 253–275.

3. McKee GK. Developments in total hip joint replacement. Symposium on lubrication and wear in living and artificial human joints. London Inst Mech Eng 1967; 85–89.
4. McKee GK, Watson-Farrar J. Replacement of arthritic hips by the McKee–Farrar prosthesis. J Bone Joint Surg 1966;48B:245–259.
5. McKee GK, Chen SC. The statistics of the McKee–Farrar method of total hip replacement. Clin Orthop 1973;95:26–33.
6. McKee GK. Development of total prosthetic replacement to the hip. Clin Orthop 1970;72:85–103.
7. Scales JT, Wilson JN. Some aspects of the development of the Stanmore total hip joint prosthesis. Reconstr Surg Traumat 1969;11:20–39.
8. Wilson JN, Scales JT. Loosening of total hip replacements with cement fixation. Clinical findings and laboratory studies. Clin Orthop 1970;72:145–160.
9. Wilson JN, Scales JT. The Stanmore metal on metal total hip prosthesis using a three pin type cup. A follow-up of 100 arthroplasties over nine years. Clin Orthop 1973;95:239–250.
10. Wilson JN, Scales JT. The Stanmore total hip prosthesis. Experience with metal to metal and metal to plastic bearings. Proceedings of the 19th World Congress of the International College of Surgeons, Lima, Peru ,1974;1:24–28.
11. Dobbs HS. Survivorship of total hip replacements. J Bone Joint Surg 1980;62B:168–173.
12. Ring PA. Complete replacement arthroplasty of the hip by the Ring prosthesis. J Bone Joint Surg 1968;50B:720–731.
13. Ring PA. Total replacement of the hip joint. A review of a thousand operations. J Bone Joint Surg 1974;56B:44–58.
14. Ring PA. Five to fourteen year interim results of uncemented total hip arthroplasty. Clin Orthop 1978;137:87–95.
15. Ring PA. Press fit prostheses: clinical experience In: Reynolds D, Freeman M (eds) Osteoarthritis in the young adult hip. Edinburgh: Churchill-Livingstone, 1989; 210–232.
16. Semlitsch M, Streicher RM, Weber H. Wear behaviour of cast CoCrMo cups and balls in long-term implanted total hip prostheses. Orthopade 1989;18:377–381.
17. Semlitsch M, Streicher RM, Weber H. Long term results with metal/metal pairing in artificial hip joints. In: Buchhorn GH, Willert HG (eds) Technical principles, design and safety of joint implants. Seattle: Hogrefe & Huber, 1994; 62–67.
18. Muller ME. Lessons of 30 years of total hip arthroplasty. Clin Orthop 1992;274:12–21.
19. Muller ME. The benefits of metal-on-metal total hip replacements. Clin Orthop 1995;311:54–59.
20. Almby B, Hierton T. Total hip replacement: a ten-year follow-up of an early series. Acta Orthop Scand 1982;53:397–406.
21. Sivash KM. The development of a total metal prosthesis for the hip joint from a partial joint replacement. Reconstr Surg Traumat 1969;11:53–62.
22. Postel M, Fayeton C. The McKee–Merle d'Aubigné prosthesis. In: Postel M, Kerboul M, Evrard J, Courpied JP (eds) Total hip replacement. Berlin: Springer, 1987; 7–9.
23. Breck LW. Preliminary report on total hip joint replacement with Urist-Thompson unit without cement. Clin Orthop 1970;72:174–176.
24. Breck LW. Metal to metal total hip joint replacement using the Urist socket. An end result study. Clin Orthop 1973;95:38–42.
25. Lunceford EM. Total hip replacement using McBride cup and the Moore prosthesis. Clin Orthop 1970;72:201–204.
26. Shorbe HB. Total hip replacement without cement. McBride acetabular component and Moore femoral prosthesis. Clin Orthop 1970;72:186–200.
27. Smith RD. Total hip replacement. Clin Orthop 1970;72: 177–185.
28. Smith RD. Total hip replacement: metal against metal. Review and analysis of cases 1961–1972. Clin Orthop 1973; 95:43–47.

29. Debeyre J, Goutallier D. Urist hip socket and Moore prosthesis without cement for hip replacement. Clin Orthop 1970;72:169–173.
30. Amstutz HC, Grigoris P. Metal on metal bearings in hip arthroplasty. Clin Orthop 1996;329S:11–34.
31. Walker PS, Gold BL. The tribology (friction, lubrication and wear) of all-metal artificial hip joints. Wear 1971;17:285–299.
32. Postel M, Arama T. The low-friction band prosthesis. In: Postel M, Kerboul M, Evrard J, Courpied JP (eds) Total hip replacement. Berlin: Springer, 1987; 9–11.
33. Schmidt M, Weber H, Schön R. Cobalt chromium molybdenum metal combination for modular hip prostheses. Clin Orthop 1996;329S:35–47.
34. McKellop H, Park SH, Chiesa R et al. In vivo wear of metal-on-metal hip prostheses during two decades of use. Clin Orthop 1996;329S:128–140.
35. Weber BG. Experience with the Metasul total hip bearing system. Clin Orthop 1996;329S:69–77.
36. Wagner M, Wagner H. Preliminary results of uncemented metal on metal stemmed and resurfacing hip replacement arthroplasty. Clin Orthop 1996;329S:78–88.
37. McMinn D, Treacy R, Lin K, Pynsent P. Metal on metal surface replacement of the hip. Clin Orthop 1996;329S:89–98.
38. Amstutz HC, Grigoris P, Dorey F. Evolution and future of surface replacement of the hip. J Orthop Sci 1998;3:169–186.
39. Amstutz HC, Sparling EA, Grigoris P. Surface and hemi-surface replacement arthroplasty. Semin Arthroplasty 1998;9:261–271.
40. Farrar R, Schmidt MB, Hamilton JV, Greer KW. The development of low wear articulations. Proceedings of the Societé Internationale de Recherche Orthopédique (SIROT) 97 Inter Meeting, Haifa, 1997.
41. Nelson K, Dyson J. Wear simulation of a metal on metal resurfacing prosthesis. Internal Publication. AEA Technology Group, Harwell, UK
42. Bobyn JD, Chan FW, Medler JB et al. Metal on metal hip testing finds less wear than in metal on polythene bearings. Orthop Int 1997;5:5.
43. McKellop H, Park SH, Chiesa R et al. Twenty-year wear analysis of retrieved metal-metal prostheses. Fifth World Biomaterials Congress, 1996, paper 854 (abstract).
44. Streicher RM, Semlitsch M, Schon RBG, Weber H, Reiker C. Metal-on-metal articulation for artificial hip joints: laboratory study and clinical results. Proc Instn Mech Engrs 1996;210:223–231.
45. Unsworth A, Dowson D, Wright V, Koshal D. The frictional behavior of human synovial joints. Part II: Artificial joints. J Lubric Tech 1975;97:377–382.
46. O'Kelly J, Unsworth A, Dowson D, Wright V. An experimental study of friction and lubrication in hip prostheses. Eng Med 1979;8:153–159.
47. Streicher RM, Schon R, Semlitsch M. Investigation of the tribological behaviour of metal-on-metal combinations for artificial hip joints. Biomedizinische Technik 1990;35:3–7.
48. Andersson GB, Freeman MA, Swanson SA. Loosening of the cemented acetabular cup in total hip replacement. J Bone Joint Surg 1972;54B:590–599.
49. Rieker CB, Kottig P, Schon R, Windler MA, Wyss UP. Clinical wear performance of metal-on-metal hip arthroplasties. In: Jacobs JJA, Craig TL (eds) Alternative bearing surfaces in total joint replacement. Philadelphia: American Society for Testing and Materials, 1988; 1346.
50. Sieber HP, Rieker CB, Köttig P. Analysis of 118 second-generation metal-on-metal hip implants. J Bone Joint Surg 1999;81B:46–50.
51. Doorn P, Campbell P, McKellop H, Benya P, Worrall J, Amstutz HC. Characterization of metal particles from metal on metal total hip replacements. 23rd Annual Meeting of the Society of Biomaterials, 1997, paper 192 (abstract).

52. Doorn P, Campbell P. Amstutz HC. Metal versus polyethylene wear particles in total hip replacements. Clin Orthop 1996;329S:206–216.

53. Green T, Fisher J, Ingham E. Polyethylene particles of a critical size are necessary for the induction of IL-6 by macrophages in vitro. 43rd Annual Meeting Orthopaedic Research Society, 1997, paper 733 (abstract).

54. Heath J, Freeman M, Swanson S. Carcinogenic properties of wear particles from prostheses made in cobalt-chromium alloy. Lancet 1971;1:564–566.

55. Meachim G, Pedley RB, Williams DF. A study of sarcogenicity associated with Co–Cr–Mo particles implanted in animal muscle. J Biomed Mater Res 1982;16:407–416.

56. Howie DW, Vernon-Roberts B. Long-term effects of intra-articular cobalt–chrome alloy wear particles in rats. J Arthroplasty 1988;3:327–336.

57. Lewis CG, Belniak RM, Plowman MC et al. Intra-articular carcinogenesis bioassays of CoCrMo and TiAlV alloys in rats. J Arthroplasty 1995;10:75–82.

58. Gillespie WJ, Frampton CM, Henderson RJ, Ryan PM. The incidence of cancer following total hip replacement [published erratum appears in J Bone Joint Surg 1996;78B(4):680]. J Bone Joint Surg 1988;70B:539–542.

59. Visuri T, Koskenvuo M. Cancer risk after McKee-Farrar total hip replacement. Orthopedics 1991;14:137–142.

60. Visuri T, Pukkala E, Paavolainen P, Pulkkinen P, Riska EB. Cancer risk after metal on metal and polyethylene on metal hip arthroplasty. Clin Orthop 1996;329S:280–289.

61. Mathiesen EB, Ahlbom A, Bermann G, Urban Lindgren J. Total hip replacement and cancer. J Bone Joint Surg 1995;77B:345–350.

62. Nyren O, McLaughlin JK, Gridley G et al. Cancer risk after hip replacement with metal implants: a population based cohort study in Sweden. J Natl Cancer Inst 1995;87:28–33.

63. Gillespie WJ, Henry DA, O'Connell D et al. Development of hematopoietic cancers after implantation of total joint replacement. Clin Orthop 1996;329S:290–296.

64. Case CP, Langkamer VG, James C et al. Widespread dissemination of metal debris from implants. J Bone Joint Surg 1994;76B:701–702.

65. Case CP, Langkamer VG, Howell RT et al. Preliminary observations on possible premalignant changes in bone marrow adjacent to worn total hip arthroplasty implants. Clin Orthop 1996;329S:269–279.

66. Jacobs JJ, Skipor AK, Doorn PF et al. Cobalt and chromium concentrations in patients with metal on metal total hip replacements. Clin Orthop 1996;329S:S256.

67. Brodner W, Bitzan P, Meisinger V, Kaider A, Gottsauner-Wolf F, Kotz R. Elevated serum cobalt with metal-on-metal articulating surfaces. J Bone Joint Surg 1997;79B:316–321.

12. Alumina on Polyethylene Bearings

L. Sedel

Introduction

John Charnley introduced metal on polyethylene (PE) articulation for total hip replacement in the early 1960s. His experience with polytetrafluorethylene (PTFE) made him acutely conscious of the problem of wear, but he estimated that this would be a mean of 0.1 mm per year, and would not represent a problem.

In 1973 Willert presented his concept of the pathophysiology of component loosening. This was essentially the consequence of the foreign body reaction to wear debris, which he documented from histological studies of retrieved tissues. As the generation of wear debris from polyethylene seemed a potential problem, other authors developed alternative bearing materials with more favourable properties.

The generation of wear debris is related to abrasive or adhesive wear. Both are directly related to surface roughness, wettability, and the chemical nature and geometry of the sphere. Scratch sensitivity and third-body wear were noted to contribute significantly to deterioration of the articular surface and were therefore a source of major concern.

Alumina ceramic was introduced to orthopaedic surgery by Pierre Boutin in 1970. He used it as a ceramic on ceramic bearing system. He and others have emphasised the smooth surface that can be obtained with this material, which together with the wettability, produces a low coefficient of friction. The main disadvantage was identified as being its brittleness, which could be overcome by using a very fine ceramic and large components. Thus, a 32-mm head size and a socket with an outer diameter of not less than 50 mm was recommended. However, it was difficult to implant these devices into small people.

This possibly explains why ceramic against PE [1] was introduced in Japan in the early eighties. Engineers worked on the tribology of ceramic on polyethylene [2-6] and they presented early interesting results showing that this combination was far superior to metal on PE with regard to the friction coefficient, wear, and resistance to third-body wear.

In this chapter we will only present information on alumina ceramic articulating with UHMWPE and not on other available ceramics such as zirconium oxide, which differs from alumina in many respects. It is a biphasic material stabilised by yttrium oxide which exhibits unusual sliding characteristics. Zirconium oxide was introduced into orthopaedic practice in 1989, and thus the clinical experience is more limited and of shorter duration.

Papers have presented reservations about properties of the material. Thus, Bragdon et al. [7] reported adverse wear properties of alumina-stabilised yttrium; however, as this material does not exist, we suspect that the authors have made an error, and attributed effects that were encountered with zirconia ceramic to alumina ceramic.

Three different aspects will now be addressed:

- the characteristics of alumina ceramics
- tribological studies
- clinical results.

Characteristics of Alumina Ceramics

Mechanical Characteristics

These mechanical characteristics include fracture toughness, sliding and wear performances, ageing and retrieval analysis.

Alumina ceramic is a stiff, hard and brittle material. It has an elastic modulus of 380 GPa compared with cobalt chromium (220 GPa), cortical bone (20 GPa) and bone cement (2 GPa). Standard alumina ceramics exhibit a bending strength of more than 400 MPa while good ceramics have a bending strength of 550 MPa.

Hardness is an important quality that determines resistance to wear. Alumina ceramic is harder than metal. Indeed, alumina ceramic is one of the hardest materials after diamonds and carborandum as determined on the Mohr scale. That is why it is used as a cutting tool in industry.

Fracture toughness

The shock sensitivity of alumina ceramics is a general source of concern. Many people believe that a brittle material will fracture under light impact loads. This is simply not true. Catastrophic failure will however result when the stress intensity factor (K_1) reaches a critical value (K_{1c}). This parameter is the fracture toughness of the material. It is determined by the direct observation of a well-defined initial crack propagation under laboratory control. Alumina ceramics have values of fracture toughness around 5 MPa $m^{1/2}$ which are lower than zirconia ceramic (9 MPa $m^{1/2}$).

To avoid excessive internal stresses the taper geometry must be accurate. This precision is required not only for the cone angle, but also for its sphericity, its roughness and its linearity. It is mandatory that the same manufacturer produces both the cone and the alumina head. Fracture resistance is related to three factors: alumina quality, cone geometry and the geometry of the inner aspect of the head. A lack of quality control and precision in any of these three areas might be responsible for subsequent fracture. In another area of concern the risk factor relates to the surgeon. Impaction of the ceramic head on the cone must be relatively smooth and gentle. It is also mandatory to avoid emergency sterilisation which involves rapid heating followed by rapid cooling. If all these requirements are met, alumina ceramic with a 32-mm diameter head on a 14/16 taper or with a 28-mm head on a 12/14 taper is a very reliable and safe material.

Laboratory tests to confirm the long-term behaviour of femoral ceramic heads involve impact tests, static strength tests and fatigue tests. Cyclical testing is generally conducted up to 10 million cycles with a load of 1.3–13.3 kN.

Head Fractures

Component fracture, and in particular head fracture, is one of the failure modes of alumina total hip arthroplasties (THAs). Because of the dramatic consequences, fracture remains one of the most important factors limiting the use of alumina couplings in clinical practice. The frequency differs from one report to another, varying from 1/1200 up to 10/130. Clinical cases of fracture have generally been associated with a small head diameter, bad quality alumina – especially a large grain size up to 40 μm – intrinsic stresses generated during the material's production, and suboptimal fitting of the male and female taper. Cement or bony fragments caught between the taper and ball do not appear to present any risk, in contradistinction to other bearing couples, including metal on metal. Improvements in the manufacturing process, taper design and greater quality control have resulted in a significant general decrease in the risk of fracture since the early 1980s. Because of these important improvements, it is difficult to estimate the exact current risk of fracture from the historical record. We reported that only one head fracture had been observed over the last ten years in more than 2000 hips. According to Clarke and Willmann [8], given that appropriate care is taken during surgery, the risk of fracture may be reduced to below 1 in 5000 cases. However, to precisely determine the fracture rate requires a prospective study over a prescribed time interval with a Kaplan–Meier analysis of the results. As relatively few series of alumina on polyethylene bearings have been reported and as this couple has only been in use for 15 years, it is difficult to determine the precise incidence of fracture with this couple. In a series of more than 60 000 total hip arthroplasties performed in the US presented by Heck et al. [9] the failure rate of the alumina ceramic head was 0.2 %.

Surface Geometry

This is an important parameter that embraces many different concepts.

Microgeometry relates not only to roughness but also to the shape of the surface irregularities. Roughness is measured by a special transducer that will give the R_a value, which is the mean height of the irregularities. It does not give the shape of these irregularities, which could be sharp or smooth. Scanning electron microscopy (SEM) examination of the surface reveals the remaining traces of machining, grain holes or any irregularities.

Macrogeometry deals with circularity which relates an equatorial plane section to a circle. Sphericity deals with circularities in every equatorial plane. When a hard material slides on a soft one, the softer will adapt to the hard one providing that the radii of curvature are not too different.

Surface Evolution with Time

Many changes will occur with articulation under load. These changes may be related to cold flow of a plastic material, to wear with the generation of debris or to surface changes not associated with the formation of debris. Some of these modifications could be considered as adaptive and part of the "bedding in" process (i.e. cold flow), but others are responsible for debris generation or severe deterioration of the surface that will compromise the function of the system.

Wear Mechanism

Wear is the mechanism by which particles of materials are released into the environment when movement occurs between two materials that are in contact with each other. These wear mechanisms are not fully understood. They are strongly influenced by the material characteristics such as hardness, modulus of elasticity, rupture behaviour, corrosion products, etc. They are also influenced by the nature and the physical characteristics of the interposed fluid – its viscosity, protein, content, pH, etc.

Four main mechanisms, which can occur simultaneously or sequentially, could describe the different wear patterns. These are adhesion, abrasion, fatigue and tribochemical.

Adhesive Wear

When two surfaces are in contact strong links called adhesive junctions are formed. When sliding starts, these junctions undergo plastic deformation and break. Four types of junction could be described: mechanical, diffusion, electronic and chemical.

- *Mechanical junction* : irregularities of the harder material penetrate into the softer one. When displacement at the interface occurs some of the soft material will remain between the irregularities of the hard one.
- *Diffusion theory*: materials may be soluble in the lubrication medium. Particles could then diffuse through the medium from one material to another. If one material is able to diffuse into the other it is known as the welding mechanism. However, if both materials are insoluble at the working temperature, the risk of diffusion is extremely low.
- *Electronic theory*: when the two counterfaces have different electronic valences, electrons could be transferred from one to another. In the case of metal against polyethylene, for example, metal gives electrons and the polymers receive them.

- *Chemical theory*: strong covalent links are generated at the interface. In the case of polymer on a metal, a metal/oxygen/carbon complex can be formed that will transfer metal onto the polymer. The predisposition of the metal to oxidise is a risk factor and of major concern. Titanium is readily oxidised, and this seems to be the reason that the wear characteristics are so poor when it articulates against polyethylene.

This adhesion mechanism is very sensitive to many parameters, such as load bearing, for example: if the load increases wear can increase dramatically. In addition, displacement speed at the interface acts on superficial temperature, which can modify the superficial structure of the plastic material. Adhesion wear is therefore a complex process influenced by many variables.

Abrasion Mechanism

This is caused by scratching or chipping of one or both surfaces. The occurrence of this type of surface damage is dependent on the mechanical characteristics of the surface – in particular, hardness and brittleness.

There are four different ways of causing abrasion: microscratching, micromachining, microchipping and microfatigue. The mechanism involved will give rise to wear debris of a different type, size, and shape. For example, chips will usually generate particles the size of the ceramic grain, while fatigue will liberate particles of a larger size.

Tribological Aspects of an Alumina on Polyethylene Couple

Alumina ceramic is an extremely interesting material, particularly with regard to its wear resistance, and this quality is related to its surface characteristics. It is possible to machine a very smooth surface finish with a R_a of 0.02, which is below the best metallic surface finish obtainable.

Its superior wear properties are also related to its ability to absorb water, which is measured by the wettability or the angle of a drop of water on its surface. This is related to the hydrophilic character of the alumina surface. This wettability could also explain the excellent friction characteristics exhibited by alumina under load [10].

Methods

Information regarding the tribological characteristics of an alumina–polyethylene couple can be obtained from different studies, including the use of simulator tests [10].

Mechanical Simulation

Two types of simulators are available: simple tribological studies involve a pin on disc or disc on disc. It is possible to run a number of these tests at the same time, but the environmental conditions are not physiological. The tests are therefore only relevant for screening, and to grossly distinguish favourable and poor materials.

The relatively sophisticated hip simulator machines are very useful. Different models are available: an attempt is made to approximate the physiological norm in the way loads and movement are applied. To understand the relevance of the information these simulators will provide, it is essential to have all the details of their design. Is the hip correctly orientated (some simulators have the acetabulum inferior)? How is the fluid distributed? Is it a closed or an open circuit? What is the running speed? What are the applied loads and what is the load cycle? How is the debris eliminated or is it contained in the sliding area? It is usually a very long and costly procedure. It is essential to know which lubricant was used (demineralised water, bovine serum, synovial fluid) as this could significantly alter the results. After the test is completed, samples are examined to provide information on wear profiles, chemical changes in the material, volume, size and type of debris, etc. Many authors have compared the function of a metal/PE couple with an alumina /PE couple [11–13]. The Al/PE couple had a lower coefficient of friction, and produced less wear. However, after 3 to 5 million cycles the coefficient of friction increases, with consequent deterioration of the articular interface. It then becomes difficult to confirm the impression of some authors that Al/PE produces five to 10 times less wear than metal/PE. A critical appraisal suggests that the real reduction in wear provided by the coupling of alumina with polyethylene is in the order of twofold.

Wear of polyethylene can be significantly influenced by alterations in the structure of the material, and by the interposition of third bodies at the interface. Medical grade polyethylene is ultrahigh molecular weight polyethylene (RCH1000). During the processing one must prevent voids or the formation of large masses of material that become organised as spherulites, as these could provide the starting point for cracks and ultimately fatigue fracture. Recently many authors have pointed out the deleterious effect of oxidation on the long-term properties of polyethylene. The resultant subsurface oxidising layer was brittle and fractured under load.

This can be avoided during sterilisation by gamma radiation in the absence of oxygen (or by alternative methods of sterilisation). The thickness of the polyethylene is critically important and catastrophic failures of the polyethylene liner were experienced with ceramic heads because of inadequate thickness of the liner [14].

Any particles of bone, cement or even hydroxyapatite will play an abrasive role [15–18]. This third-body wear mechanism might be responsible for early wear of polyethylene material [19]. One of the major advantages of ceramic could be to reduce this third-body wear. Alumina ceramic surfaces are not as sensitive to scratching or pitting as metallic surfaces are. This, however, presents another potential complication: after fracture of an alumina head or revision of alumina components, some alumina debris may remain. If at revision surgery the alumina head is replaced by a metallic one, these alumina particles could remain in the polyethylene (or indeed in the surrounding tissues) and then give rise to severe damage of the metallic femoral head with consequent catastrophic wear of the polyethylene [20]. It is therefore strongly advocated that an alumina ceramic material is always replaced by another ceramic in order to avoid such complications.

During simulation tests the temperature in the polyethylene can rise while it remains stable in the metal. This rise in temperature could be associated with some adverse effects. Bergmann et al. [21] measured a temperature elevation in vivo in humans during walking. This could clearly play a role in the degradation process of the materials.

Effects of the Counterface Material

Abrasive wear as well as fatigue are observed with alumina ceramic on PE but not before 500 km. The phenomenon usually started somewhere between 1000 to 4000 km of the test. Some authors have emphasised the different effects caused by the design of the sliding tests. For example, unidirectional tests gave better results for ceramic on polyethylene than reciprocating tests [22]. Moreover the sensitivity of the tests was influenced by the nature of the fluid film. For example, Al/PE is less influenced by bovine serum or demineralised water than metal/PE. In contradistinction to other authors [23, 24] they also found 40% less wear with zirconia heads than with alumina heads. Moreover alumina on polyethylene demonstrated a lower coefficient of friction in bovine serum than in demineralised water – in which it increased with the length of the running time [23].

Clarke et al. studied the effects of the size of the ceramic head on the friction coefficient [25]; 22-mm heads appeared to do better than 28-mm heads.

Clarke compared alumina on polyethylene and alumina on alumina in a recent paper [26]. He concluded that alumina on polyethylene produced 600 times more wear as determined by hip simulator studies and from analysis of retrieved explants.

Clinical Results

The alumina/PE clinical experience started in the early 1980s, some 10 years later than ceramic on ceramic, and there are thus few long-term clinical results available. Early clinical results were published by Willert and Zichner in Germany [27, 28] Schuller [29] and Sugano [30].

Jenny et al. [3] reported on the French clinical experience from seven different centres and reviewed 1347 total hip arthroplasties performed in patients younger than 50 years of age. They compared the incidence of aseptic loosening or osteolysis using different friction couples. They could find no statistically significant differences in the incidence of the osteolysis or aseptic loosening between alumina on PE and metal on PE. The only demonstrable difference was that alumina on alumina exhibited statistically less osteolysis than the other couples.

In the paper by Sugano [30], 61 total hips were implanted in 54 patients from 1981 to 1983. The mean age was 53 years (31–70). Fifty-seven hips were followed up for a mean of 11.1 years (10–13). The Merle d'Aubigné score revealed 77% to be good. Radiological loosening occurred in three femoral components and 16 acetabular components. Wear of the socket was in the order of 0.1 mm per year. However a higher rate of wear was observed in the early postoperative years than later on. A high rate of wear correlated with calcar resorption (P 0.002), but not with acetabular loosening. Study of retrieved implants showed excellent surface roughness, sphericity and bending strength of the heads. However, scratches and voids were observed on the sockets. Comparable results have been published in Germany. In a sequential study the same surgical technique was used to insert the same prosthesis with a standard head size: the composition of the head was the only variable. At a 10-year follow-up the revision rate for alumina/PE was 30% less than with metal/PE [27]. In a more recent study [28] the authors reported on socket penetration comparing ceramic and metal heads. Ceramic exhibited an initial penetration rate in the order of 0.5 mm per year. However, after 5 years this penetration rate diminished to 0.1 mm for the ceramic compared with 0.2 mm for the metal. Wear/penetration of more than 0.2 mm per year is considered unfavourable

and associated with a higher incidence of loosening of the prosthesis. In a series of 369 total hip prostheses, the ceramic/polyethylene combination was noted to produce half of the total amount of wear produced by metal/polyethylene.

Le Mouel et al. [31] reported a series of 156 alumina on polyethylene prostheses implanted from 1983 to 1985 in 131 patients. The 10-year survivorship was 93.5% with revision from whatever cause (sepsis, recurrent dislocation or aseptic loosening) as the endpoint. No aseptic loosening or osteolysis of the femoral stem was encountered. An 8-year follow-up by the same surgeons of the same stem design with two different friction couples revealed a 79% survivorship for the metal on polyethylene against 97.6% for the alumina on polyethylene. However, once again, this was a cohort and not a randomised study.

We have implanted more than 400 prostheses with an alumina on polyethylene couple since 1983 (Fig. 12.1). We have not encountered a fracture of the femoral head. Some sockets demonstrated quite marked early wear, but this was non-progressive. There have been no retrievals, although several hips have been lost to follow-up. It should be noted that this series has a built-in bias as these prostheses were only implanted into older patients, an alumina/alumina couple being used for the younger, more active patient. It is, therefore, not possible to make a direct comparison.

We now use 28-mm alumina heads and an all-polyethylene cemented socket. Over the past 5 years economic constraints in health care have dictated that we use both metallic and alumina heads.

Simon et al. [14] reported on catastrophic failure of a polyethylene liner resulting in the ceramic head penetrating the metal shell with a resultant massive foreign body reaction. We have encountered a similar complication on two occasions (Fig. 12.2). We therefore strongly advocate that an all-polyethylene socket – and not a metal-backed implant – be used with a ceramic head.

Oonishi et al. [5] analysed retrieved polyethylene prostheses explanted after periods of 2 to 7 years of clinical use. The average in vivo wear rate of polyethylene articulating against 28 mm alumina heads was reported as 0.1 mm per year.

Fracture of the alumina head when coupled with polyethylene has rarely been reported in clinical practice. This could be ascribed to the relatively recent use of this couple with improved alumina ceramic material. McKellop et al. [32] presented some unusual fracture rates which may be attributed to a fault in the design of the Morse taper. Hummer et al. [1] reported on catastrophic failure of zirconia ceramic femoral heads.

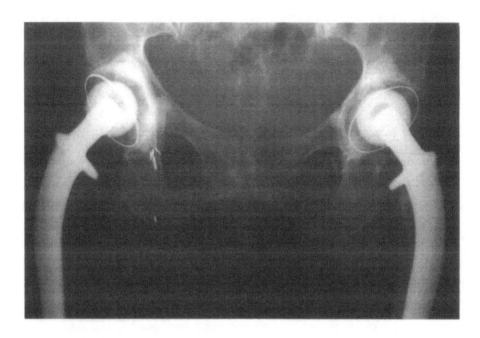

Fig. 12.1.   Radiological aspects after 13 years (R) and 7 years (L) in a 72-year-old woman. Clinical results are excellent on both sides.

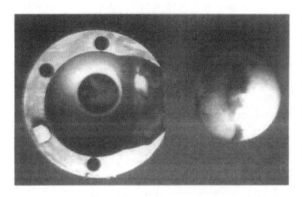

Fig. 12.2.   Complete wear out of a metal-backed polyethylene socket. The alumina head ruined the titanium alloy shell after only 4 years.

Conclusion

The Al/PE couple exhibited superior tribological characteristics compared with metal on PE. However, this improvement is not easy to quantify. Laboratory tests suggest that the amount of wear debris could be reduced by a factor of 2. Some clinical results have revealed a significantly lower incidence of aseptic loosening of prostheses incorporating this couple.

We believe that the major advantage of ceramic is related to the improved resistance to third body wear. This will increase the durability of the implant by reducing the amount of wear debris that is generated. However, the generation of even a limited amount of wear debris remains a potential problem in the long term. As this will be strongly influenced by the longevity of implantation and the activity level, we still recommend alumina on alumina in active young patients, and, as suggested by Black [33], reserve alumina on polyethylene for the less active, middle-aged patient.

References

1. Hummer CD 3rd, Rothman RH, Hozack WJ. Catastrophic failure of modular zirconia-ceramic femoral head components after total hip arthroplasty. J Arthroplasty 1995;10(6):848–850.
2. Dorlot JM. Long-term effects of alumina components in total hip prostheses. Clin Orthop 1992;282:47–52.
3. Jenny JY, Boeri C, Tavan A, Schlemmer B. Résultats en fonction du couple de frottement. In: Symposium sur les prothèses totales de hanche avant 50 ans (Directeurs: L Pidhorz et L Sedel) Revue Chir Orthop 1998; Suppl1, 84:75–120.
4. Kawauchi K, Kuroki Y, Saito S et al. Total hip endoprostheses with ceramic head and HDP socket. Clinical wear rate. In: Oonishi H and Ooi Y (eds) Orthopaedic ceramic implants. Japanese Society of Orthopaedic Ceramic Implants, 1984;4:253–257.
5. Oonishi H, Takayaka Y, Clarke I, Jung H. Comparative wear studies of 28-mm ceramic and stainless steel total hip joints over 2 to 7 year period. CRC press. J Long-term Effects M Implants 1992;2(1):37–47.
6. Davidson JA. Characteristics of metal and ceramic total hip bearing surfaces and their effect on long-term ultra high molecular weight polyethylene wear. Clin Orthop 1993;294:361–378.
7. Bragdon CR, Jasty M, Kawate K et al. Wear of retrieved cemented polyethylene acetabula with alumina femoral heads. J Arthroplasty 1997;12(2):119–125.

8. Clarke IC, Willmann G. Structural ceramics in orthopedics. In: Cameron HE (ed) Bone implant interface. St. Louis, MO: Mosby, 1994; 203–252.

9. Heck DA, Partridge CM, Reuben JD, Lanzer WL, Lewis CG, Keating EM. Prosthetic failures in hip arthroplasty surgery. J Arthroplasty 1995;10:575–580.

10. Dumbleton JH, Miller DA. A simulator for load bearing joints. Wear 1972;20:165–174.

11. McKellop HM, Clarke IC, Maelkorf KL, Amstutz HC. Friction and wear properties of polymer metal and ceramic prosthetic joints materials evaluated on a multichannel screening device. J Biomed Mat Res 1981;15:619–653.

12. Wroblewski BM, Siney PD, Dowson D, Collins SN. Prospective clinical joint simulator studies of a new total hip arthroplasty using alumina ceramic heads and cross-linked polyethylene cups. J Bone Joint Surg 1996;78B, 280–285.

13. Sedel L. Tribology of total hip replacement. Instructional Course Lecture. EFORT meeting, Barcelona, 1997. Edited by P Fulford and J Duparc.

14. Simon JA , Dayan AJ, Ergas E, Stuchin SA, Dicesare PE. Catastrophic failure of the acetabular component in a ceramic-polyethylene bearing total hip arthroplasty. J Arthroplasty 1998;13(1):108–113.

15. Caravia L, Dowson D, Fischer J, Jobbins B. The influence of bone and bone cement debris on counterface roughness in sliding wear tests of ultra high molecular weight polyethylene on stainless steel. Eng Med 1990;204:65–70.

16. Cooper JR, Dowson D, Fisher J, Jobbins B. Ceramic bearing surfaces in total artificial joints resistance to third body wear damage from bone cement particles. J Med Eng Technol 1991;15(2):63–67.

17. Isaac GH, Arkinson JR, Dowson D, Kennedy PD, Smith MR. The causes of femoral head roughening in explanted Charnley hip prostheses. Eng Med 1987;16(3):167–173.

18. Weightman BO, Swanson SAV,Isaac GH, Wroblewski BM. Polyethylene wear from retrieved acetabular cups. J Bone Joint Surg 1991;73B(5):806–881.

19. Davidson JA, Poggie RA, Mishra AK. Abrasive wear of ceramic, metal and UHMWPE bearing surfaces from third-body bone, PMMA bone cement, and titanium debris. Biomed Mater Eng 1994;4(3):213–229.

20. Kempf I, Semlith M. Massive wear of a steel ball head by ceramic fragments in the polyethylene acetabular cup after revision of a total hip prosthesis with fractured ceramic ball. Arch Orthop Trauma Surg 1990;109(5):284–287.

21. Bergmann G, Graichen F, Rohlmann A. In vivo measurement of temperature rise in a hip implant. Proceedings 37th Annual Meeting Orthopaedic Research Society, Anaheim, USA, 1991; 223.

22. Kumar P, Oka M, Ikeuchi K et al. Low wear rate of UHMWPE against zirconia ceramic (Y-PSZ) in comparison to alumina ceramic and SUS 316L alloy. J Biomed Mater Res 1991;25(7):813–828.

23. Boher C. Simulation experimentale du comportement tribologique des matériaux prothétiques de la hanche. Thèse en sciences des matériaux, Toulouse, 1992.

24. Streicher RM, Semlitsch M, Schön R. Ceramic surfaces as wear partners for PE. In: Bonfield W, Hastings GW, Tanner KE (eds) Bioceramics 4 (Proceedings of the 4th International Symposium on Ceramics in Medicine), London, 1991; 9–16.

25. Clarke IC, Gustafson A, Jung H, Fujisawa A. Hip-simulator ranking of polyethylene wear: comparisons between ceramic heads of different sizes. Acta Orthop Scand 1996;67(2): 128–132.

26. Clarke IC. Optimal wear performance of ceramic on ceramic bearings for THR. Proc Annual Japanese Joint Arthroplasty. Kanazawa, Japan, 1998; 1, In press.

27. Zichner LP, Willert HG. Comparison of alumina–polyethylene and metal–polyethylene in clinical trials. Clin Orthop 1992;282:86–94.

28. Zichner L, Lindenfeld T. In vivo wear of the slide combinations ceramic–polyethylene as opposed to metal-polyethylene. Orthopade 1997;26(2):129–134.

29. Schuller HM, Marti RK. Ten-year socket wear in 66 arthroplasties. Ceramic versus metal heads. Acta Orthop Scand 1990;61(3):240–243.

30. Sugano N, Nishii T, Nakata K, Mashura K, Takaoka K. Polyethylene sockets and alumina ceramic heads in cemented total hip arthroplasty. A ten year study. J Bone Joint Surg 1995;77B (4):548–556.

31. Le Mouel S, Allain J, Goutallier D. Analyse actuarielle à 10 ans d'une cohorte de 156 prothèses totales de hanche cimentées à couple de frottement alumine/polyethylene. Rev Chir Orthop 1998;84(4):338–345.

32. McKellop HA, Sarmiento A, Brien W, Park SH. Interface corrosion of a modular head total hip arthroplasty. J Arthroplasty 1992;7(3):291–294.

33. Black J. Metal on metal bearings, a practical alternative. Clin Orthop 1996;329S:244–255.

13. Ceramic on Ceramic Bearing Surfaces

J. Witvoet, R. Nizard and L. Sedel

Introduction

The principal cause of aseptic loosening of total hip arthroplasty (THA) in the mid and long term is caused by the reaction of the periprosthetic bone to wear particles both from the components of the implanted prosthesis (metal, polyethylene, ceramic, carbon, etc.), and from cement if cement is used. Wear debris occurs at the head-socket interface even if the prosthesis is securely fixed, and movement between prosthesis and bone is limited.

The metal–polyethylene couple and the ceramic–polyethylene couple are the two most frequently used head socket combinations. Friction between two materials will often result in wear of the less durable material – polyethylene in this case.

The polyethylene debris – which consists of submicron particles – is ingested by macrophages, and activates local inflammatory mediators (cytokines, interleukins, etc.) leading to periprosthetic osteolysis, which in turn leads to loosening of the components of the prosthesis in the medium to long term.

Figure 13.1 provides a typical example of this phenomenon. At 12 years follow-up the prosthesis on the right side demonstrates minimal wear of the polyethylene and shows no sign of loosening while the one on the left shows severe plastic wear with loosening of the acetabular component. This phenomenon occurs in both cemented and cement-less protheses. It is indeed possible to minimise the wear of the polyethylene by improving the surface of the metallic head (i.e. with ion bombardment), improving the quality of the polyethylene, or by using ceramic femoral heads. However, the fact remains that the longer the prosthesis remains in situ the greater the likelihood of polyethylene wear, particularly if the patient is heavy and active.

It was for this reason that other head socket couples were used. The metal–metal couple used in the 1960s and 1970s in the McKee–Farrar and Ring prostheses – probably the most widely known – was associated with a high incidence of early loosening. This could be ascribed to the high frictional torque which compromised the fixation of the implant. As a result metal on metal was abandoned at one stage but has again been introduced in recent years with encouraging results.

Advantages and Disadvantages of the Alumina–Alumina Couple

In 1970 the French orthopedic surgeon Pierre Boutin was the first to use a ceramic–ceramic coupling; this was an alumina–alumina couple. The components are made out of a vacuum-packed aluminum powder compressed at very high temperature. This coupling has three distinct advantages:

1. The coefficient of friction between the surfaces is low and does not degrade with time. This is mainly due to the wettability of the alumina (Fig. 13.2) [1–2].
2. Many authors have demonstrated that the wear of an alumina–alumina coupling is minimal [1–3]. Dorlot [3] has estimated that it is 4000 times less than in a metal–polyethylene coupling. Indeed, Dorlot has analysed explants and shown that the average wear was 0.025 μm per year.
3. The wear particles of the alumina excited a limited inflammatory response – as demonstrated

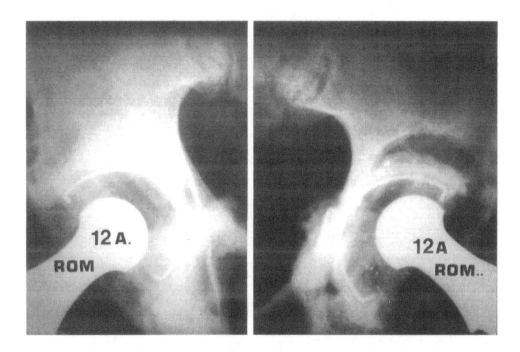

Fig. 13.1. Twelve years follow-up of two Charnley low friction arthroplasties. Right: no wear, no loosening; left: PE wear and aseptic loosening of the cup.

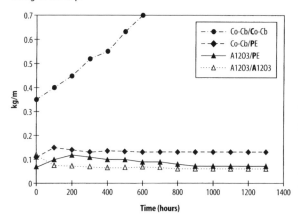

Fig 13.2. Different friction couples on a hip simulator.

Fig. 13.3 Importance of clearance, circularity and sphericity in alumina–alumina bearing surfaces.

by Willert, Lerouge and Sedel [1, 6–8]. This is due to the fact that alumina is an inert material.

The identified advantages of an alumina–alumina coupling can be obtained only when:

(i) the alumina is of sufficiently high quality, and
(ii) tight tolerances are maintained in the manufacture of the bearing surfaces between the femoral head and the acetabulum (Fig. 13.3).

The quality of the alumina must meet the requirements of international standards (Table 13.1) the most important of which include the average size of the alumina crystals (< 3 μm), the roughness and the sphericity coefficient of the two components.

The contact surface of the two components must be as great as possible, and the clearance produced by the different radii of the head and of the cup must be less than 10 μm. Disregard of this important aspect perhaps explains the significant wear that some surgeons initially observed with the use of the alumina–alumina coupling.

In our experience, from 1977 to 1990 the two articulating components were matched and non-interchangeable. Today the manufacture of this alumina–alumina coupling allows interchangeability of the two pieces. Finally, it is imperative that the acetabular component is not implanted too vertically (45°

Table 13.1. Specifications of Ceraver alumina component

A1$_2$O$_3$	> 99.8%
SiO$_2$ and other oxides	< 0.05%
Density (g/cm^3)	> 3.93
Microhardness (Vickers)	23 000
Compressive strength (MPa)	4500
Bending strength (MPa)	550
Young's modulus (GPa)	380
Fracture toughness (MPa In)	5–6
Average grain size (μm)	3–4
Surface finishing Ra (μm)	0.02

off vertical is optimal) as this reduces the bearing surface. Dorlot [3] has reported severe wear associated with tilting of the acetabular component.

Given the advantages of the alumina–alumina coupling, it seems surprising that its use is so limited in the world. There are two reasons for this. The first is the brittleness of the alumina. Head fractures [4, 9–11] were reported quite frequently in the 1970s, due both to the difficulty of manufacturing consistently high quality material, and to problems associated with the method of fixation of the head on the metallic stem.

We commenced using an alumina–alumina couple in 1977, and had three fractures of the head in 1978. One occurred with a 22-mm head used with a very small cup in a congenital dislocation (this size is no longer used). In the other two cases 32-mm heads were used and a manufacturing defect was subsequently detected. Since 1978 we have encountered only one head fracture, which occurred following a car accident, in over 3000 alumina heads. One incomplete fracture of the acetabular component was noted in a patient with recurrent dislocation.

Fritch and Gleitz [9] reported only one fracture from 1763 implanted femoral heads (0.06%). In addition to the quality of the alumina, the method of fixation of the head on the femoral stem is an important factor. Fixation utilising a Morse taper trunion is the only accepted method at this time. Some femoral heads with a collar – such as the Mittelmeier prostheses [8] – have been associated with a higher percentage of fractures as a result of impingement of the ceramic collar against the acetabular component. The geometry of the Morse taper must correspond exactly to the inner geometry of the ceramic head. It is hazardous to combine a femoral head and a Morse taper from two different manufacturers, as the specifications may not be precisely matched. It is also important to protect the Morse taper and avoid scratching at the time of implantation, and to clean it thoroughly prior to application of the head.

It is essential that heavy hammering is avoided when the head is impacted onto the trunion. Despite the use of gentle impaction we have never encountered a case of head/neck disassembly, even in hips with recurrent dislocation. These well-established operative precautions must be adhered to.

Description of the Prosthesis

We have used an alumina–alumina coupling in our department since 1977. It should be noted, however, that financial considerations prevent us from using this coupling on all implanted prostheses. The coupling is only used for very active patients with a life expectancy of over 10 years. In the other patients, a metal–polyethylene coupling is used in conjunction with an all-polyethylene cemented cup with established excellent results in which the implant will generally outlast the patient.

The Osteal Ceraver prosthesis (Fig. 13.4) is composed of an alumina–alumina coupling and a titanium alloy cemented femoral stem. The femoral component, which has not changed since 1977, is modular, the ceramic head being fixed by a Morse taper. The fixation of the cup has evolved since 1977 (Fig. 13.5). Between 1977 and 1982, the cup was cemented. Between 1983 and 1989, the cup was modular, with a screw-threaded titanium alloy (TA6V4) shell and an alumina insert which was fixed by an inverted Morse taper. From 1990 to 1998 a modular press-fit acetabular component was used. The titanium alloy shell was covered by a pure titanium mesh which promoted osseo-integration. The mesh is securely fixed by rivets and peripheral rings, which do not interfere with the mechanical properties and characteristics of the metal-backed cup. The rationale for these modifications in the fixation mode of the cup will be further explained during discussion of the clinical results.

Clinical and Radiological Results

Cemented Alumina–Alumina Prosthesis [10– 12, 14–16]

Between 1977 and 1983 we implanted 600 cemented alumina–alumina prostheses, 401 of which were primary hip arthroplasties. Only the results of the primary interventions will be discussed.

The primary pathology was coxarthrosis or light dysplasia in 88.1%, while only 3.15% had rheumatoid arthritis. The average age was 63.5 years: 55.8% were females and 44.5% males. Review at 12 months

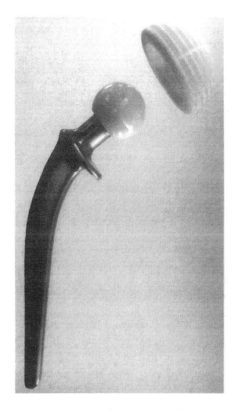

Fig. 13.4 Ceraver osteal alumina–alumina hip prosthesis.

or more was not available on 55 hips. Only the results of the 345 hips followed up for more than one year will be presented (Fig. 13.6). The mean follow-up was 10 years. The clinical results assessed by the Postel–d'Aubigné score were 85.7% very good and good, 2.4% fair and 11.9% poor.

These poor results related to 48 loose acetabular components: only six hips had associated loosening of the femoral component (1.5%). The 10-year survival using the Kaplan–Meier survival analysis with aseptic loosening as the endpoint (Fig. 13.7) was 86.4% (85.9–92.9%) for the cup and 98.1% (96.2–100%) for the femoral stem. The 15-year survival was 78.1% (71.5–84.5%) for the cup and 97.3% (94.4–99.8%) for the femoral stem. The mechanism of loosening of the 48 acetabular components was virtually identical in every instance, with debonding between the cement and the alumina cup (Fig. 13.8).

A finite element analysis study by Crolet et al. [17] demonstrated that the difference in elasticity between the cement and the cup was responsible for this "debonding". This led to the microfractures of the cement, with consequent resorption of the bone in contact with the cement. Finally a total fracture of the cement occurred from the upper iliac segment down to the posterior ischiopubic region. This

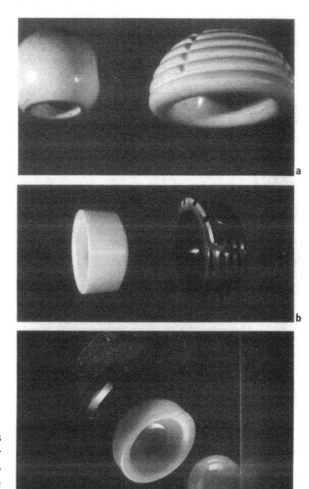

Fig. 13.5 Different modes of Ceraver cup fixation: **a** cemented cup; **b** screw-in cup; **c** press-fit cup.

explains why the method of fixation of the cup was modified in 1983. On the other hand, the excellent long-term results of the femoral component (with 14 different sizes) persuaded us to continue with the same cemented implant.

Alumina–Alumina Prosthesis with a Screw-in Cup (Fig. 13.5)

The encouraging results of screw-in cups which were published around this period influenced us to choose this mode of fixation for the cup. The component was composed of a cylindrohemispherical shell of titanium alloy into which an alumina core was fixed by an inverted taper. From 1984 to 1990, 430 screw-in cups were implanted at primary arthroplasty. The average age was 61.7 (± 12 years). The pathology

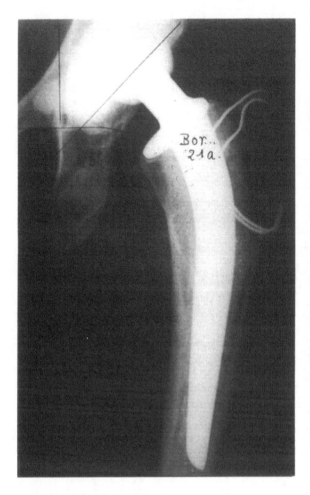

Fig.13.6. All cemented alumina–alumina Ceraver THA at 21 years follow-up.

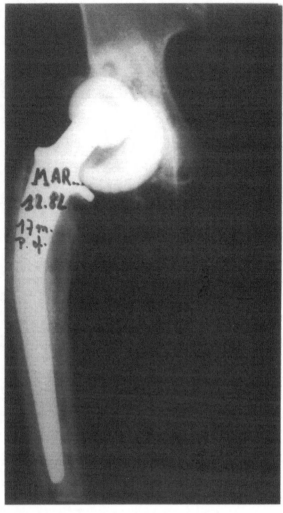

Fig. 13.8. Mechanical loosening by debonding between the cement and the alumina cup.

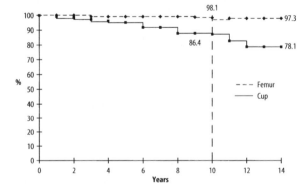

Fig. 13.7. Survival curve (Kaplan–Meier) for cemented cup and femoral stem (endpoint: aseptic loosening).

was osteoarthritis in 70%, developmental dysplasia of the hip (DDH) in 19.3%, osteonecrosis in 7% and only 1% rheumatoid arthritis. All of the patients had been followed up for more than one year. The average follow-up was 8.2 years (1–4 years). The clinical results (Fig. 13.9) assessed using the Postel-Merle d'Aubigné system were: 90.7% very good and good results, 5.6% fair results, while 3.7% were regarded as failures.

The radiological results were unfortunately less encouraging for the acetabular component. According to the criteria of Engh and Massin [18], 48 cups were judged to have migrated. Of these 17 have been revised because of severe pain. This high incidence of migration has been widely reported, and is attributed to the very smooth external surface of the implant rather than to the use of alumina and not polyethylene as the bearing articular surface. However, among these 430 prostheses only one case of aseptic femoral loosening has been encountered (0.23%) and only one perifemoral osteolysis (in a

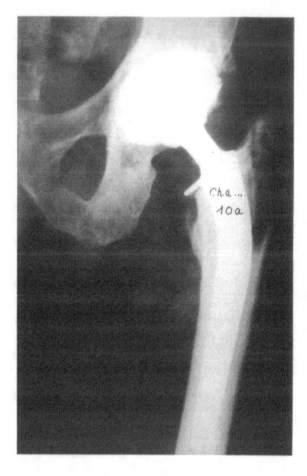

Fig. 13.9. Screw-in alumina–alumina cup Ceraver THA at 10 years follow up.

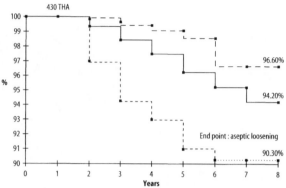

Fig. 13.10. Survival curve (Kaplan–Meier) for primary screw-in cup (endpoint: aseptic loosening).

single zone of Gruen and Amstutz) [19]. The actuarial survival curves with aseptic loosening as the endpoint reveal the screw-in cup to have a survival rate of 94.3% at 8 years (Fig. 13.10).

Alumina–Alumina Prosthesis with a Press-fit Cup (Fig. 13.5)

Concern about the 31 cups that had migrated and had not yet been revised persuaded us to change the method of fixation of the acetabular component. From 1990 a press-fit hemispherical titanium alloy shell covered with a coating of pure titanium mesh was used. The fixation of the mesh to the shell has been modified (rivet and peripheral ring fixation) on the latest models. The alumina insert was secured with a reverse Morse taper similar to that used with the screw-threaded cup.

Of these prostheses, 709 were inserted between 1990 and 1997. To ensure an adequate follow-up only the 259 prostheses inserted in 239 patients between

1990 and 1993 were reviewed. There were 137 males and 122 females: 20 patients had bilateral arthroplasties. The average age was 59.5 (± 11.8 years) with an average weight of 71.4 kg (± 16.5 kg) and an average height of 1.66 m (± 9.1 cm).

The primary pathology was osteoarthritis or mild DDH in 84%, and osteonecrosis in 9.3% with only 1.9% rheumatoid arthritis. Twenty-five patients were lost to follow-up or had further surgery within 1 year (one for septic arthritis and one for recurrent dislocation). Two hundred and thirty-four hips were followed up for more than one year with a mean of 3.2 years (range 1–7 years). The clinical results (Fig. 13.11) were assessed according to the Postel–Merle d'Aubigné system: 95.9% were regarded as good, 2.8% as fair and 1.3% as failures. These three failures correspond to three cases of aseptic loosening that occurred between 3.5 and 5 years. Of these, two were attributable to a failure of fixation of the early press-fit cup, while debonding of the pure titanium mesh from the substrate accounted for the third. There was only one case of aseptic loosening of the femoral component.

The radiological appearances at the last follow-up were quite reassuring. There were only 23 acetabular lucent lines, 19 of which were in Delee–Charnley zone 3, and two in both zone 2 and zone 3. Two cases had a lucency in all three zones but these were only 1 mm in width and were non-progressive. There was no sign of peri-acetabular osteolysis. Eight femoral radiolucent lines were observed and all were confined to a single zone (zone 5). The actuarial survival curve with aseptic loosening as the endpoint at 6 years follow-up was 97.9% for the acetabular component and 99.8 % for the femoral component (Fig. 13.12).

Conclusions

More than 20 years experience using a total hip replacement composed of a cemented titanium alloy femoral component and an alumina–alumina couple has permitted us to draw the following conclusions:

1. The wear of the alumina–alumina friction couple in vivo reproduces the laboratory findings (wear hip simulator testing). Thus, minimal wear was encountered as long as high quality alumina was used, and the appropriate clearance produced by the differing radii of the two components was maintained.
2. Fracture of the components is extremely rare. This is true for the femoral head as long as the Morse taper of the femoral stem is matched with the femoral head (the heads are not interchangeable from one manufacturer to another).
3. The cemented titanium alloy femoral stem used in our department has been used continuously without modification and has given excellent long-term results.
4. Loosening of the acetabular component was always a mechanical problem, both with the cemented alumina cup and with the modular screw-in cup.
5. The use of a modular press-fit cup since 1990 has greatly reduced the problems of fixation of an alumina bearing to the iliac bone. It is hoped that the fixation will remain durable.
6. Periprosthetic osteolysis, which is a major long-term complication of prostheses using a metal polyethylene couple, was virtually not encountered (two cases from 1139 hybrid hip replacements) when alumina couplings were used.
7. The alumina–alumina couple is considerably more expensive than a metal–polyethylene or an alumina–polyethylene couple. Its use has therefore been reserved for active patients with good bone stock and a life expectancy of more than 10 years.
8. For older patients or those with a low activity profile, excellent results have been obtained with the same cemented femoral stem combining a metal– or alumina–polyethylene couple with an all-polyethylene cemented cup.

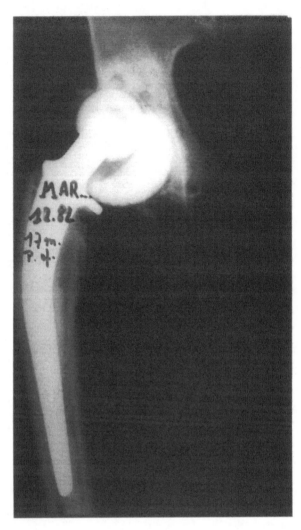

Fig. 13.11. Press-fit alumina–alumina cup Ceraver THA at 7 years follow up.

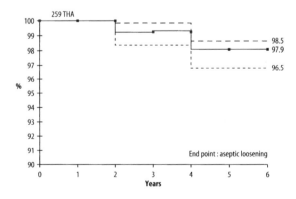

Fig. 13.12. Survival curve (Kaplan–Meier) for primary press-fit cup (endpoint: aseptic loosening).

References

1. Taylor SK, Serekian S, Monley M. Wear performance of a contemporary alumina–alumina friction couple under anatomically relevant hip joint simulator. Poster at the 65th AAOS meeting, New Orleans, 1998.
2. Walter A. On the material and the tribology of alumina–alumina coupling for hip joint prostheses. Clin Orthop 1992;282:31–47.

3. Dorlot JM (1992) Long-term effect of alumina components in total hip prostheses. Clin Orthop 282:47–53

4. Willmann G. Oxide ceramics for articulating components of total hip replacement. Proceedings of the 10th International Conference on Ceramics in Medicine, Paris. Bioceramics 1997;10:123–130.

5. Christel P. Biocompatibility of surgical grade dense polycrystalline alumina. Clin Orthop 1992;282:10–19.

6. Lerouge S, Huk O, Yahia L, Sedel S, Witvoet J. Ceramic-ceramic on metal–PE. A comparison of periprosthetic tissue from loosened total hip arthroplasty. J Bone Joint Surg 1997;79B:135–139.

7. Lerouge S, Huk O, Yahia L, Sedel S. Characterisation of in vivo wear debris from ceramic-ceramic total hip arthroplasty. J Biomed Mater Res 1996;32:627–633.

8. Willert HG, Semlitsch M. Reactions of the articular joint capsule to wear products of artificial joint prostheses. J Biomed Mater Res 1977;11: 157.

9. Fritsch EW, Gleitz M. Ceramic femoral head fractures in THA. Clin Orthop 1996;328:129–136.

10. Higuchi F, Shiba N, Inone A, Wakebe I. Fracture of an alumina ceramic head in total hip arthroplasty. J Arthroplasty 1995;10:851–854.

11. Nizard R, Sedel L, Christel P, Meunier A, Soudry M, Witvoet J. Ten years survivorship of cemented ceramic-ceramic total hip prostheses. Clin Orthop 1992;282:53–64.

12. Plenk H, Buhler M, Walter A, Knahr K, Salter M. Fifteen years experience with alumina ceramic total hip joint endoprostheses: a clinical, historical and tribological analysis. In: Ravagliolo A, Krewski A (eds) Bioceramic and the human body. Amsterdam: Elsevier Science, 1992; 17–25.

13. Quack G, Willenamm G, Pieper H, Krall H. Improvement of THR with spongiosa metal surface using the wear couple ceramic on ceramic. Proceedings of the 10th International Symposium on Ceramics in Medicine, Paris. Bioceramics 1997;10:123–130.

14. Mittelmaier H, Heisel J. Sixteen years experience with ceramic hip prostheses. Clin Orthop 1992;282:64–73.

15. Sedel L, Nizard R, Kerboull L, Witvoet J. Alumina–alumina hip replacement in patients younger than 50 years old. Clin Orthop 1994;298:175–184.

16. Winter M, Griss P, Scheller G, Moser T. Ten to 14 years results of a ceramic hip prosthesis. Clin Orthop 1992;282:73–81.

17. Crolet JM, Christel P, Sedel L, Witvoet J. Comparative numerical simulation of humaniliae bone fitted with different types of acetabular component (0.20 finite elements analysis). 4th European Conference on Biomaterials, 1983.

18. Massin P, Schmidt MD, Engh CA. Evaluation of cementless acetabular component migration. J Arthroplasty 1989;4(3) 245–251.

19. Gruen TA, McNeice GM, Amstutz HC. "Modes of failure" of cemented stem-type femoral components: a radiographic analysis of loosening. Clin Orthop 1979;141:17–27.

Section VI

Infected Interface

14. Periprosthetic Infection – Bacteria and the Interface Between Prosthesis and Bone

L. Frommelt

Introduction

Medical advances over the last decades have made it possible to implant devices to support physiological functions, such as pacemakers, or replace natural anatomical sites, such as total joint replacements or vascular prostheses. On the other hand, many temporary indwelling devices, such as intravenous catheters, are in common use. All these indwelling medical devices are at the risk of being colonised by microbes and may even lead to life-threatening infection [3–6]. Nowadays physicians are therefore confronted with infections due to the implantation of foreign materials into a human body – so-called biomaterial-associated infections. This was alarmingly demonstrated by artificial hearts: almost all devices became severely infected during the first 90 days after implantation and had to be removed [1, 2].

Implant-associated infections are characterised (as stated by Gristina, Naylor and Myrvic [10]) by: "(1) adhesive bacterial colonisation; (2) a biomaterial or damaged tissue substratum; (3) resistance to host defence mechanisms and antibiotic therapy; (4) the presence of characteristic bacteria such as *Staphylococcus epidermidis*, *Staphylococcus aureus* and *Pseudomonas aeruginosa*; (5) the transformation of non-pathogens or opportunistic pathogens into virulent organisms by the presence of a biomaterial substratum; (6) frequent polymicrobial infections; (7) persistence of the infection until the substratum is removed; and (8) the absence of adequate tissue integration at the biomaterial/tissue interface."

A common characteristic of the different biomaterials and devices used is that they interact like bacterial pathogens with host defence mechanisms and that there are specialised bacteria that are able to colonise the foreign body's surface. The susceptibility to bacterial colonisation varies according to the materials used [5, 7].

In alloarthroplasty, the location where the interaction between the biomaterial and the recipient's individual defence takes place is the space between the surface of the prosthesis and the bone: *the interface*. If bacteria are involved, periprosthetic infection occurs on the surface of the prosthetic device. Understanding the interaction between foreign materials and bone, between bacteria and the biomaterial's surface and between bacteria and the host defence – all taking place at the interface – is the key to understanding periprosthetic infection.

Bacterial Pathogens and Host Defence

Man and bacteria live together in a state of "truce" rather than in "peace". Several species inhabiting the surfaces of the human anatomy are well-known pathogens when transported to other sites of the body, e. g. *E. coli* from the gut to the urinary bladder. If bacteria succeed in invading a new environment they cause an infection at the moment when the host reacts to the invader. Whether infectious disease occurs depends on the efficacy of the host defence and on the virulence of the pathogen. High-grade pathogens such as *Salmonella typhi* are usually able to overwhelm the host defence. The outcome of infectious disease is either the death of the host or elimination of the pathogen. The most important mechanism of elimination is phagocytosis by

macrophages and polymorphonuclear (PMN) leucocytes in blood and tissue. Without phagocytosis no
antimicrobial agent is able to stop an infectious
disease by elimination of the bacterial pathogen. As
long as the pathogen is present, the host defence
produces an inflammatory reaction leading to
phagocytosis, e.g. by macrophages.

If elimination of bacterial pathogens does not
occur and the infection does not lead to the death
of the host, it may culminate in the formation of
granuloma, as in tuberculosis. Macrophages meta-
morphose into epitheloid cells and giant cells that
surround the area of necrosis containing the
pathogen and induce fibroblasts to form connective
tissue. Finally, encapsulation of the bacteria occurs
and they become invisible to host defence. In the
centre of such a lesion *Mycobacterium tuberculosis*
may survive for decades without doing any harm to
the host, but the bacteria are also resistant to attack
by the host.

Bacteria and Interfaces

Understanding micro-organisms requires an understanding of their environmental conditions and
recognising that bacterial life is determined by the
ability to adapt to their environment. The environment of bacterial life can consist of liquid, gaseous
and solid materials, which may be organic or inorganic. Bacteria interact with these different materials
whether they are part of a living organism or not. If
the environment consists of a mixture of several
materials, the same bacterial strain may occur in the
several different conditions produced at the interface where the bacteria are living. It is estimated that
surfaces submerged in a stream of water can be
colonised by approximately 10^6 bacteria/ml, whereas
the water contains 10^2 to 10^3/ml. Bacteria are bound
to the surfaces by a fine network of polysaccharide
fibres [8]. Any discontinuity in an environmental
system creates a "surface", or better, an interface,
which is capable of modifying the composition of
the bacterial population [9]. These interfaces are
formed – as noted by Brisou [9] – by solids/liquids,
solids/gases, and non-miscible fluids such as water/
hydrocarbons, water/oils, etc. It should be pointed
out that all these interfaces have surfaces to which
bacteria can stick by various mechanisms.

The interface prosthesis/bone tissue is regarded
by bacteria as two different interfaces, one to the
bone tissue and one to the foreign material.

From Adsorption to Biofilm: Micro-organisms and Solid Interfaces

Microbiologists study bacteria under optimised
conditions in the laboratory that do not reflect the
life of bacteria living "in the wild". Bacteria are culti-
vated in optimised nutrient media at an optimal pH
and temperature. Under these conditions they are
able to reproduce in about 30 minutes. Millions of
bacteria are held in pure cultures in order to study
their physiological properties and their susceptibility
to several antimicrobial agents. In most situations
this, together with the complaints of the patient,
represents a good method of characterising the
bacterial pathogen and providing suggestions for
antimicrobial therapy to the physician which will
have good predictive value. In cases with damaged
tissue or in the presence of indwelling medical
devices this no longer holds true. Bacteria causing
periprosthetic infection are partially in a state of
adherence to a foreign body surface and partially in
a vegetative state causing infectious disease in the
surrounding tissue.

Bacteria adhering to foreign bodies are part of a
complex ecological system, the biofilm. The biofilm
bacterium differs fundamentally from the planktonic
cell of the same species. Adhesion triggers the
depression of a large number of genes, which leads
to a modified phenotype which resembles a dormant
state or incomplete sporulation [9,19].

Surfaces: Attraction and Adhesion of Bacteria

Brisou [9] states that the process of bacteria
becoming closely bonded to surfaces is divided into
three steps: (1) adsorption mediated by the physic-
ochemical properties of surfaces; (2) adhesion, a
specific mechanism of stereochemical molecular
recognition; and (3) adherence, a state in which
bacteria are anchored to a surface by the formation
of biofilm. The first two steps , adsorption and adhesion, are completely reversible, whereas adherence
is an irreversible state of bacterial bonding to a
surface.

Bacteria may reach the surface in several states,
most often as free-living germs in an aquatic environment, which with few exceptions in nature represents a colloidal solution. In this state they can be
adsorbed to a surface by mechanisms that are caused
by physicochemistry. Hydrophobic attraction, Van
der Waals' forces, and electrostatic attraction are
often the first mediators of adsorption of bacteria to

the surface [1, 9]. This is consistent with a theory developed by Derjarguin and Landau [11] and Verwey and Overbeek [12] (as quoted by [9, 13]), which is called the DLVO theory according to the authors' initials; immersed objects have the tendency to attract other objects to their surface. The DVLO theory states that there are two thermodynamic states near a surface in a colloidal solution:

1. Forces that act at long range (1–10 mm from the surface) and are composed of a variety of weak forces that attract particles such as gravitation, electrostatic attraction, Van der Waals' forces, and surface tension.
2. Forces that act at short range (less than 1 mm from the surface) that are both repulsive and attractive. Of these Van der Waals' forces and steric configurations repel particles, whereas hydrophobic, covalent, hydrogen, and ionic bonding attract particles [1, 10]. Due to these bivalent mechanisms, adhesion is a reversible state.

Polycations such as amino acids, calcium ions, ferric ions and others play an important role in overcoming the electrostatic repulsion between bacteria which are negatively charged on their surface and also from which substratum surfaces are negatively charged. These ions are characterised by more than one positive loading, which enables them to abolish the repelling forces between bacteria and substratum, which may be not only an inorganic substratum but also more highly organised cells or even micro-organisms.

Bonding to receptors is another more specific way to manage adhesion, especially at the surface of cells or mediated by glycoproteinaceous residue, the conditioning film on the surface of passive substrata. Theoretically, this docking to receptors is reversible, but in most cases bacterial anchorage organelles act almost simultaneously or with a short delay. This leads directly to irreversible adherence by so-called adhesins.

Bacterial Adhesins and Formation of Biofilm

In the 1950s many fundamental studies were carried out to investigate the structure of bacterial cells, their organelles, and their envelope. Later, attention was directed at a special function of these structures – the adherence of bacteria. This is crucial to produce virulence and thus pathogenesis of infectious disease. Bacterial adhesins are molecules or organelles on the microbial surface that are able to bind the bacterial cell to a surface [14]. The outer surface of micro-organisms is formed by the bacterial capsule covering the bacterial cell wall in which bacterial organelles are anchored. The organelles are fibrillae, fimbriae (i.e. Pili 1), sexual pili, and, if present, flagella. Of these, fimbriae play an important role in binding bacteria to surfaces. These fimbriae are looked upon as structural lectins, molecules which manage a selective binding to cells showing certain carbohydrate patterns. Another important mechanism of binding bacteria to surfaces is mediated by the glycocalyx, a superficial polysaccharide containing structure on the external surface of cells in general[15]. Sutherland [16] noted that the bacterial cells are able to form glycocalyx as well. Glycocalyx appears as slime which acts as a sort of glue [17]. It has two functions: (1) intrinsic glycocalyx is necessary for the viability of cells; (2) extracellular glycocalyx is not necessary for viability but forms a crucial part of biofilm [18, 19].

Eukaryotic cells are able to mediate adherence by membrane receptors that bind protein in a typical receptor–ligand fashion [21]. These mechanisms are not only relevant for bacterial adherence but also for the integration of foreign materials. What is needed to colonise passive substrata is a conditioning film of protein debris [22, 35] that allows bacteria to stick and furthermore enables fibronectin or laminin, for example, to promote bacterial binding [23–25].

The final state of adherence is a biofilm formed by vast amounts of slime substances harbouring bacterial microcolonies well protected from dehydration and attacks from the host defence. In nature, these biofilms are mostly inhabited by more than one bacterial species. It is a complex microbial community with a primitive homeostasis, a primitive circulatory system, and metabolic co-operation [19]. The biofilm bacteria differ in phenotype from the planktonic form of the same species: adherence in biofilm leads to suppression of a large number of genes as, for example, the expression of antibiotic susceptibility patterns. Bacteria living in biofilm are more resistant to antibacterial agents. The doubling time is dramatically prolonged: Zak [26] found propagation cycles of more than 20 hours in *Staphylococcus aureus* from bone sequestra. Since antimicrobial agents take effect only during reproduction of metabolically active bacteria, this behaviour deprives antibiotics of their usual locus of action. Together with the genetic alteration described by Costerton and associates [19, 28, 31, 32, 34] it seems impossible to cure infection of foreign material by systemic antibiotic therapy.

Another effect of biofilm is due to the slime itself. The extracellular slime is able to inhibit the antimicrobial action of glycopeptide antibiotics[27]. The slime of *Pseudomonas aeruginosa* is able to act as a diffusion barrier to some antibiotics, e.g. piperacillin

[33]. Furthermore, the slime acts on host defence mechanisms, especially on the phagocytotic activity of PMN leucocytes [29, 30]. The slime also interferes with the action of the macrophage, which is one of the principal cells in host defence [32].

The mechanisms of adherence vary from species to species and are best recognised in staphylococci and *Pseudomonas aeruginosa*. Even the adhesins of different species show a vast molecular variety with respect to structure, expression, and biological activity [36]. This may be of advantage when competing for a special ecological niche in the biofilm, which in nature is often inhabited by several types of micro-organisms.

In periprosthetic infection biofilm represents a reserve where bacteria are separated from the host's inner environment and defence mechanisms. Furthermore, the bacteria change their phenotypic appearance by genetic regulation so that antibiotics lose their target while, as noted, the slime itself is able to interfere with the cellular defence of the host.

Foreign Bodies Inside the Human Body

Both foreign bodies and bacteria are recognised by the host defence as foreign. Both micro-organisms and foreign materials induce a reactive inflammation and both elicit the same response: macrophages and PMN leucocytes incorporate foreign material and try to degrade these materials by enzymatic release from cellular organelles. However, foreign bodies often cannot be eliminated by enzymatic digestion. In these cases macrophages play a crucial role. They induce a specific morphological lesion, the foreign body granuloma – as in tuberculosis. This condition occurs when a foreign body is too large to be ingested and removed even by giant cells varying from 10 – 100 μm in diameter. The foreign body then induces macrophages to stimulate fibroblasts to form granulation tissue. Finally the foreign body is encapsulated by a tight, dense membrane of connective tissue [37]. In artificial joint replacement slight interfacial motion is associated with resorption and remodelling of the bone bed, activation of macrophages and production of wear particles followed by formation of an interfacial membrane. The quiescent interfacial membrane is composed of a thin layer of connective tissue, as in granulomas. This membrane does not necessarily interfere with the biological function of the implant [38]. Both mechanical and chemical factors can influence the outcome. Even biomaterials regarded as "inert" can be the source of many chemical irritants able to induce and perpetuate a chronic inflammation[37]. Gristina [39] describes an immuno-incompetent fibro-inflammatory zone surrounding biomaterial implants featuring cellular damage and susceptibility to bacterial infection. This zone may induce a self-perpetuating inflammatory response which corresponds to the lytic interfacial membrane described by Boss and associates [38]. However, this interfacial membrane serves as the immunological frontier between the host and the biomaterial implant. Due to the fact that this membrane itself is immuno-incompetent, bacteria may induce periprosthetic infection if they succeed in reaching this area, e.g. by the bloodstream. On the other hand, bacteria that had colonised the biomaterial previously are protected by the interfacial membrane and can act undisturbed by the host defence mechanisms.

The Interface: The Key Element in Biomaterials with Regard to Infection vs. Integration

The interface between prosthesis and bone is the place where the future of an artificial joint replacement is decided. Integration of the foreign material is a complex process that results in a stable situation regarded by host defences as a no-man's land where biomaterials, and bacteria if present, are undisturbed by mechanisms intended to eliminate foreign substances (including bacteria). If toxic substances are released from the biomaterial a chronic inflammatory response mediated by macrophages with the tendency for self-perpetuation may occur and lead to loosening of the prosthesis. If the inflammatory process comes to an end without extensive osteolysis a thin interfacial membrane will remain which does not interfere with biomechanical properties of the prosthetic device.

The interfacial membrane consists of connective tissue originating from fibroblastic activity. A point of particular interest is that cellular colonisation of a surface with either fibroblasts or bacteria is mediated by glycocalyx. This leads to what Gristina called "a race for the surface" between bacteria, if present, and fibroblasts [1, 2]. If fibroblasts have already settled, bacteria will fail to colonise, and vice versa.

Colonisation alone however does not cause an infection or an infectious disease. If bacteria succeed in colonising a prosthetic device it often takes quite a long time for periprosthetic infection to become established. In our own experience more than 50% of the deep infections of artificial joint replacements occurring within a period of 10 years became manifest during the first year after implantation. This can be explained by the fact that adherent bacteria hidden in biofilm spread by slow continuous growth along the surface of the biomaterial and by dispersion provoked by micromovement in the interface. Biofilm and the organisation of the interface, as noted above, prevents the host defence from interacting with these bacteria. The periprosthetic infection does not become established until the bacteria leave the biofilm and the interface and induce local osteomyelitis. The consequence of this is that less virulent micro-organisms may be disguised for months or even years.

Normally, bacteria spread around the surface of the prosthesis over a long period of time, so that wide areas have been covered by the time clinical symptoms occur. In this context it should be noted that the synovial fluid does not act as a barrier to bacteria. If periprosthetic infection becomes established at any location, all components of an artificial joint replacement have to be considered as infected.

Bacterial Specialists in Colonising Surfaces

Even though attachment and adhesion is a general survival strategy of bacteria [9, 10] the ability to use these mechanisms depends on the specific characteristics of each bacterium and the conditions found at the interface. Some micro-organisms, like *Mycobacterium tuberculosis*, seem to have no specific mechanisms to stick to biomaterials [40]. Others, like staphylococci, are able to adhere in small numbers [44] and use adhesins formed by the host like fibronectin, lamellin, and others [25, 41, 47]. In coagulase-negative staphylococci the explicit mechanism of virulence derives from its excellent ability to adhere to surfaces [42, 43].

Some *Staphylococcus aureus* strains have special mechanisms for creating a bond to bone and connective tissue [45, 46, 51], which are of relevance in osteomyelitis, septic arthritis, and in periprosthetic infection as well.

Curiously, only a few species are predominantly involved in the pathogenesis of infection of indwelling devices. *Staphylococcus epidermidis* and *Staphylococcus aureus* are the most frequently isolated germs from biomaterial surfaces [3, 10, 48, 50] but other micro-organisms like propionibacteria, β-haemolytic streptococci, corynebacteria, *Pseudomonas aeruginosa*, enterobacteriaceae and others may be involved in periprosthetic infection.

The range of bacterial species encountered in these infections is not only due to the ability of the specific micro-organisms to adhere to the bio-material used, but also which bacteria are present at the probable site of infection.

Origin of Bacteria in Periprosthetic Infection

Bacterial pathogens are theoretically able to reach the prosthetic device in three ways: (1) direct contamination during the surgical procedure either from the patient's own flora or from contaminated air in the operating room; (2) through the bloodstream with bacteriaemia or septicaemia; or (3) by continuous spread from an adjacent infection – erysipelas, for example.

As noted by Lidwell, over 95 % of periprosthetic infections occurring during the first year after artificial joint replacement are due to intraoperative colonisation of the prosthesis by contaminated air [52, 53]. It has to be presumed that direct contamination of bacteria from the patient's skin is also relevant. Brown and co-workers [55] point out that air contamination results not only from the type of ventilation but also from the activity in an operating room with ultra-clean air. In conclusion, direct contamination of the biomaterial derives both from the flora of the patient and to a certain extent from the skin of the operating team. In these infections bacteria inhabiting the human skin predominate. This is confirmed by the bacteria isolated in our own series[50] (Table 14.1).

This contamination does not only occur in artificial joint replacement but also in all other procedures performed in an operating room. However, in other fields of surgery, the number of these bacteria is too small to cause infection as they are rapidly eliminated by the host defence. If a foreign body is involved the situation is totally different: a very small number of less virulent micro-organisms are able to colonise the foreign body surface and cause an early periprosthetic infection.

The haematogenous origin is relevant for infections that occur later, but these are encountered less frequently [54]. Here the pathogen is transported from a distant site of infection by the bloodstream or by lymphatic vessels to the prosthesis. Bartzokas and associates [56] convincingly exposed the relation between infections of the teeth and subsequent infection of an artificial joint replacement.

Table 14.1. Bacterial isolates responsible for periprosthetic infection: 1077 isolates listed by rank (ENDO-KLINIK, Hamburg, 1985–1989)

No.	Type of bacteria	Number	Percentage
		(absolute; $n =$)(%)	
1	*Staphylococcus epidermidis / spp.*	441	41.95
2	*Staphylococcus aureus*	282	26.18
3	*Propionibacterium* spp.	93	8.64
4	*Steptococcus* spp.	66	6.13
5	*Peptostreptococcus* spp.	44	4.09
6	*Pseudomonas aeruginosa*	40	3.71
7	*Enterococcus* spp.	24	2.23
8	*Corynebacterium* spp.	15	1.39
9	*Escherichia coli*	11	1.02
10	*Candida albicans*	9	0.84
11	*Proteus* spp.	8	0.74
12	*Bacteroides* spp.	6	0.56
13	*Enterobacter* spp.	6	0.56
14	*Klebsiella* spp.	5	0.46
15	*Serratia* spp.	5	0.46
16	*Haemophilus influenzae*	5	0.46
17	*Mycobacterium* spp.	5	0.46
18	*Salmonella* spp.	3	0.28
19	*Clostridium* spp.	3	0.28
20	*Citrobacter* spp.	2	0.19
21	*Listeria monocytogenes*	2	0.19
22	*Veillonella* spp.	1	0.09
23	not identified	1	0.09
	Organism 1 + 2		68.13
	Organism 1 – 4		82.90
	Organism 5 – 23		17.10

Approach to the Therapy of Periprosthetic Infection with respect to Pathogenesis

Bacteria sticking to the surface of a biomaterial are well protected against host defence by biofilm and against antibiotics by several mechanisms. The latter depend partly on the bacterial species involved. Biofilm produced by *Pseudomonas aeruginosa* acts as a diffusion barrier because of the presence of alginate in the biofilm [19, 28, 31, 34]. Even though this mechanism was thought to be present in other types of bacteria it does not exist in most species, and therefore has to be considered as an exception. In staphylococci and most other bacteria a diffusion barrier does not exist, but another mechanism is present: extended time of reproduction [19, 26]. Because antimicrobial agents act only when bacteria are multiplying, antibiotics lose their target. Further-

more, antibiotics are not able to eliminate bacteria without the assistance of a cellular defence which will kill bacteria by phagocytosis. Phagocytically active cells like macrophages and PMN leucocytes are inhibited in the presence of biofilm. Encapsulation to a granuloma, as described above, also acts to prevent phagocytotic cells from carrying out their function.

Under these conditions systemic antibiotics will fail to eradicate bacteria submerged in biofilm, but bacteria which have left the biofilm to induce local osteomyelitis, for instance, can be influenced by the antimicrobial agents. The situation is well known to physicians: all parameters of an infection will disappear, sinuses will close, and biochemical signs of infection will decrease. The infection is suppressed but not cured. After antibiotic therapy has ceased the infection will start again, originating from the surface of the prosthesis.

The only exceptions are acute infections with a virulent pathogen which manifest shortly after implantation. These can be treated in the early stages of becoming established on the foreign body surface. In such cases therapy by suction drainage together with systemic antimicrobial therapy as recommended by Mella-Schmidt and Steinbrink [57] or systemic therapy with a combination of chinolones and rifampicin as proposed by Zimmerli and co-workers [58, 59] may be successful.

In all other cases the removal of the prosthesis is crucial for the outcome of periprosthetic infection [3, 50, 60, 61]. From the point of view of a specialist in infectious diseases, it is not important whether the procedure is one-stage, two-stage, or revision with removal of the prosthesis. The essential point is that in all described methods of revision the foreign body has to be removed completely. Surgical intervention has to be radical and debridement has to include all infected bone and soft tissue and all components of foreign material of the joint replacement.

In the case of two-stage revision cement spacers impregnated with suitable antibiotics should be used. Exceptions to this are infections with yeast. To date there is no known antifungal agent that can be eluted from bone cement. In our experience, however, one-stage revision is possible if performed in combination with systemic therapy with amphotericin B and flucytosin.

Conclusions

The pathogenesis of periprosthetic infection is a complex process in which the interface between bone and artificial joint replacement is not only the site where the infection occurs, but also the key area in the understanding of the complex interactions between the host, the biomaterial, and the pathogens.

The host defence acts against biomaterial and bacterial pathogens in a similar way: if elimination is impossible, bacteria and biomaterial are separated by a granuloma-like lesion and are thus to some extent protected from further attacks by the host defence. The morphological substratum is connective tissue and the interfacial membrane, which is normally a quiescent zone, does not interfere with the biomechanical properties of the prosthetic device. However, if irritated by movement in the interface or chemically by debris from biomaterial, it changes into a chronic self-perpetuating inflammatory state. This is the immuno-incompetent fibroinflammatory zone as described by Gristina, and is a precursor of aseptic loosening of the prosthesis. In this state the interface is quite susceptible to bacterial colonisation and subsequent periprosthetic infection.

If bacteria are present in the substance of the interfacial membrane, there will be competition between bacteria and fibroblasts in colonising the foreign material: the so-called race for the surface. This occurs as both bacteria and fibroblasts have similar mechanisms for colonisation using glycocalyx and peptidoglycans produced by cells, including those of prokaryotes.

If bacteria succeed in colonising the surface of the foreign body they will establish a new primitive ecological system, the biofilm. Biofilm as a general strategy of survival protects bacteria from environmental influences and, in the special situation of indwelling medical devices, from the attack of host defence mechanisms and from the effect of antimicrobial agents. What results is double protection of the colonising bacteria, and it seems likely that the immuno-incompetent fibro-inflammatory zone derived from the interfacial membrane enables bacteria to leave the interface and induce infection of adjacent tissue. It is unclear whether the bacteria play a role in the transformation of the interfacial membrane to a chronic inflammatory state.

The type of reaction that occurs at the interface is also influenced by the biomaterial. Being "inert" means that a biomaterial provokes only a slight reaction by the host defence which leads to the formation of a quiescent interfacial membrane. Fibroblasts are then able to colonise the biomaterial easily, which in turn leads to integration. In most materials this results in a situation where bacteria have the same advantages as tissue cells.

Unfortunately, it is rather confusing that the process is not controlled by a strict hierarchy and it is therefore not possible to predict what will happen next, as the interactions between host, biomaterial, and bacteria are both quantitative and qualitative. Action and reaction occur simultaneously and not synchronously in all parts of the surfaces involved. Undesired reactions may lead to a chain reaction which becomes self-perpetuating and culminates in the failure of the prosthesis whether it is infected or not.

In periprosthetic infection the point of no return is closely related to adherence, the irreversible state of bacterial binding to a biomaterial surface with subsequent colonisation. Unfortunately, the number of bacteria necessary for colonising biomaterial surfaces is small so that minimal contamination will lead to colonisation if the bacteria become adherent.

What can be done is to avoid contamination whenever possible, and if contamination is inevitable, to prevent pathogens from colonising the foreign material. This can be achieved by mixing antibiotics with the bone cement. This is effective, because the antimicrobial agents act directly at the presumed site of infection before the prosthesis becomes colonised.

Other strategies include looking for biomaterials that have a limited interaction with the host defence and are thus able to slow down reactions in the interfacial membrane in order to avoid irreversible self-perpetuating reactions which lead to failure of the arthroplasty. The challenge is well articulated by Gristina: "Biomaterial surfaces must be modified to improve compatibility and tissue integration and to resist microbial contamination in the race for the surface."

Acknowledgements

I thank K. Schreyer, B.A. for her excellent support in writing this article in a foreign language.

References

1. Gristina AD. Biomaterial-centred infection: microbial adhesion versus tissue integration. Science 1987;237:1588–1595 .
2. Gristina AD, Dobbins JJ, Giammara B, Lewis JC, DeVries WC. Biomaterial-centered sepsis and total artificial heart: microbial adhesion vs tissue integration. JAMA 1988; 259:870–874.
3. Buchholz HW, Elson RA, Engelbrecht E, Lodenkämper H, Röttger J, Siegel A. Management of deep infection of total hip replacement. J Bone Joint Surg 1981;63B:342–353.
4. Eftekhar NS. Long-term results of cemented total hip arthroplasty. Clin Orthop 1987;225:207–217.
5. Ludwicka A, Locci R, Jansen B, Peters G, Pulverer G. Microbial colonization of prosthetic devices: V. Attachment of coagulase-negative staphylococci and "slime"-production on chemically pure to synthetic polymers. Zbl Bakt Hyg I.Abt Orig B 1983;177:527–532.

6. Khardori N, Yassien M. Biofilms in device-related infections. J Ind Microbiol 1995;15:141–147.

7. Oga M, Sugioka Y, Hobgood CD, Gristina AG, Myrvic QN. Surgical biomaterials and differential colonization by *Staphylococcus epidermidis* Biomaterials 1988;9:285–289.

8. Roth JL. The lectin molecular: probes in cell biology and membrane research. Jena: Fischer, 1978.

9. Brisou JF. Biofilms – methods of enzymatic Release of micro organisms. Boca Raton: CRC Press, 1995.

10. Gristina AG, Naylor PT, Myrvik QN. Biomaterial-centered infections: microbial adhesion versus tissue integration. In: Wadström T, Eliasson I, Holder I, Ljungh A (eds) Pathogenesis of wound and biomaterial-associated infections. London: Springer, 1990; 193–216.

11. Dejaguin BV, Landau L. Theory of the stability of strongly charged lyophilic sols and the adhesion of strongly charged particles in solutions of electrolytes. Acta Physiochem URSS 1941;14:633–656.

12. Verwey EJW, Overbeek JTG. Theory of stability of lyophobic colloids. London: Elsevier, 1948.

13. Baddour LM, Christensen GD, Simpson WA, Beachey EH. Microbial adherence. In: Mandell GL, Douglas RG jr, Bennett JE (eds) Principles and practice of infectious diseases, 3rd edn. New York: Churchill Livingstone, 1990;. 9–25.

14. Duguid JP. Fimbriae and adhesive properties in *Klebsiella* strains. J Gen Microbiol 1959;21:271–286.

15. Bennet HS. Morphological aspect of extracellular polysaccharides. J Histochem Cytochem 1963;11:14–23.

16. Sutherland IW. Bacterial exopolysacherides – their nature and production. In: Sutherland IW (ed.) Surface carbohydrates of the prokaryotic cell. London: Academic Press, 1977.

17. Costerton JW, Geesey GG, Cheng K-J. How bacteria stick. Sci Am 1978;238:86–95.

18. Ito S (1969) Structure and function of the glycocalyx. Fed Proc 28:12–25

19. Costerton JW, Lewandowski Z, Caldwell DE, Korber DR, Lappin-Scott HM. Microbial biofilms. Ann Rev Microbiol 1995;49:711–745.

20. Gristina AG, Naylor PT, Myrvik QN. Molecular mechanisms of musculoskeletal sepsis. In: Esterhai JL, Gristina AG, Poss R (eds) Musculoskeletal infection. Park Ridge: American Academy of Orthopedic Surgeons, 1992; 13–28.

21. Vercelotti GM, McCarthy JB, Lindholm P, Peterson PK, Jacob HS, Furcht LT. Extracellular matrix proteins (fibronectin, laminin, and type IV collagen) bind and aggregate bacteria. Am J Pathol 1985;120:13–21.

22. Williams RL, Williams DF. The spatial resolution of protein adsorption on surfaces of heterogeneous metallic biomaterials. J Biomed Mater Res 1989;23:339–350.

23. Nylor PT, Ruch D, Brownlow C, Webb LX, Gristina AG. Fibronectin binding in orthopedic biomaterials and its subsequent role in bacterial adherence. Trans Orthop Res Soc 1989;14:561–564.

24. Daroiche RO, Landon GC, Patti JM et al. Role of *Staphylococcus aureus* surface adhesins in orthopaedic device infections: are results of model-dependent? J Med Microbiol 1997;46: 75–79.

25. Hermann M, Vaudaux PE, Pittet D et al. Fibronectin, fibrinogen, and laminin act as mediators of adherence of clinical staphylococcal isolates. J Infect Dis 1988;158: 693–701.

26. Zak O, Sande MA. Correlation of in vitro activity of antibiotics with results of treatment in experimental animal models and human infection. In: Sabath LD (ed.) Action of antibiotics in patients. Bern: Hans Huber Publishers, 1982; 55–67.

27. Farber BF, Kaplan MH, Clogston AG. *Staphylococcus epidermidis* extracted slime inhibits the antimicrobial action of glycopeptide antibiotics. J Infect Dis 1990;161:37–40.

28. Arizono T, Oga M, Sugioka Y. Increased resistance of bacteria after adherence to polymethylmethacrylate. Acta Orthop Scand 1992;63:661–664.

29. Johnson GM, Lee DA, Regelmann WE, Gray ED, Peters G, Quie PG. Interference with granulocyte function by *Staphylococcus epidermidis* slime. Infect Immun 1986;54:13–20.

30. Zimmerli W, Lew PD, Waldvogel FA. Pathogenesis of foreign body infection – Evidence for a local granulocyte defect. J Clin Invest 1984;73:1191–1200.

31. Webb LX, Holman J, de Araujo B, Zaccaro DJ, Gordon ES. Antibiotic resistance in staphylococci adherent to cortical bone. J Orthop Trauma 1994;8:28–33.

32. Myrvik QN, Wagner W, Barth E, Wood P, Gristina AG. Effects of extracellular slime produced by *Staphylococcus epidermidis* on oxidative responses of rabbit alveolar macrophages. J Invest Surg 1989;2:381–389.

33. Hoyle BD, Alcantara J, Costerton JW. *Pseudomonas aeruginosa* biofilm as a diffusion barrier to piperacillin. Antimicrob Agents Chemother 1992;36:2054–2056.

34. Khoury AE, Lam K, Ellis B, Costerton JW. Prevention and control of bacterial infections associated with medical devices. ASAIO J 1992;38:M174–178.

35. Francois P, Vaudaux P, Foster TJ, Lew DP. Host-bacteria interactions in foreign body infections. Infect Control Hosp Epidemiol 1996;17:514–520.

36. St.Geme JW 3rd. Bacterial adhesins: determinants of microbial colonisation and pathogenicity. Adv Pediatr 1997;44: 43–72.

37. Coleman DL, King RN, Andrade LD. The foreign body reaction: a chronic inflammatory response. J Biomed Mater Res 1974;8:199–211.

38. Boss JH, Shajrawi I, Mendes DG. The nature of the bone–implant interface. The lessons learned from implant retrieval and analysis in man and experimental animal. Med Prog Technol 1994;20:119–142.

39. Gristina AG. Implant failure and the immuno-incompetent fibro-inflammatory zone. Clin Orthop 1994;298:106–118.

40. Oga M, Arizono T, Takasita M, Sugioka Y. Evaluation of the risk of instrumentation as a foreign body in spinal tuberculosis. Clinical and biologic study. Spine 1993;18: 1890–1894.

41. Herrmann M, Lai QJ, Albrecht RM, Mosher DF, Proctor RA. Adhesion of *Staphylococcus aureus* to surface-bound platelets: Role of fibrinogen/fibrin and platelets integrins. J Infect Dis 1993;167:312–322.

42. Peters G, Pulverer G. Pathogenesis and management of *Staphylococcus epidermidis* "plastic" foreign body infections. J Antimicrob Chemotherap 1984;14(Suppl. D):67–71.

43. Peters G. New considerations in the pathogenesis of coagulase-negative staphylococcal foreign body infections. J Antimicrob Chemother 1988;21(Suppl. C):139–148.

44. Zimmerli W, Waldvogel A, Vadeau P, Nydegger UE. Pathogenesis of foreign body infections: description and characteristics of an animal model. J Infect Dis 1982;146:487–497.

45. Ryden C, Maxe I, Franzen A, Ljungh A, Heinegard D, Rubin K. Selective binding of bone matrix sialoprotein to *Staphylococcus aureus* in osteomyelitis. Lancet 1987;ii:515.

46. Speziale P, Raucci G, Visai L, Switalski LM, Timpl R, Hook M. Binding of collagen to *Staphylococcus aureus* Cowan 1. J Bacteriol 1986;167:77–81.

47. Mohammad SF, Topham NS, Burns GL, Olsen DB. Enhanced bacterial adhesion on surfaces pretreated with fibrinogen and fibronectin. Trans Am Soc Artif Intern Organs 1988; 34:573–77.

48. Christensen GD, Simpson WA, Beachey EH. Adhesion of bacteriato animal tissue: complex mechanisms. In: Savage DC, Fletcher M (eds) Bacterial adhesion: mechanisms and physiologic significance. New York: Plenum Press, 1985; 279–305.

49. Gristina AG, Hobgood CD, Barth E. Biomaterial specificity, molecular mechanisms and clinical relevance of *S. epidermidis* and *S. aureus* infections in surgery. In: Pulverer G, Quie PG, Peters G (eds) Pathogenesis and clinical significance of coagulase -negative staphylococci. Stuttgart: Fischer, 1987; 143–157.

50. Steinbrink K, Frommelt L. Behandlung der periprothetischen Infektion der Hüfte durch einzeitige Austauschoperation. Orthopäde 1995;24:335–343.

51. Symersky J, Patti JM, Carson M et al. Structure of the collagen-binding domain from a *Staphylococcus aureus* adhesin. Nat Struct Biol 1997;4:833–838.

52. Lidwell OM, Lowbury EJ, Whyte W, Blowers R, Stanley SJ, Lowe D. Effect of ultraclean air in operating rooms on deep sepsis in the joint after total hip or knee replacement: a randomised study. Br Med J (Clin Res Ed) 1982;285:10–14.

53. Lidwell OM, Lowbury EJ, Whyte W, Blowers R, Stanley SJ, Lowe D. Infection and sepsis after operation for total hip or knee-joint replacement: influence of ultraclean air, prophylactic antibiotics and other factors. J Hyg (Lond) 1984;93:505–529.

54. Gillespie WJ. Infection in total joint replacement. Infect Dis Clin North Am 1990;4:465–484.

55. Brown AR, Taylor GJ, Gregg PJ. Air contamination during skin preparation and draping in joint replacement surgery. J Bone Joint Surg Br 1996;78B:92–94.

56. Bartzokas CA, Johnson R, Jane M, Martin MV, Pearce PK, Saw Y. Relation between mouth and haematogenous infection of total joint replacements. BMJ 1984;309:506–508.

57. Mella-Schmidt C, Steinbrink K. Stellenwert der Spül-Saug-Drainage bei der Behandlung des Frühinfektes von Gelenkimplantaten. Chirurg 1989;60:791–794.

58. Zimmerli W. Die Rolle der Antibiotika in der Behandlung der infizierten Gelenkprothese. Orthopäde 1995;24:308–313.

59. Zimmerli W, Zak O, Vosbeck K. Experimental hematogenous infection of subcutaneously implanted foreign bodies. Scand J Infect Dis 1985;17:303–310.

60. Wagner H, Wagner M. Infizierte Hüftgelenksprothese. Gesichtspunkte für den einzeitigen und zweizeitigen Prothesenwechsel. Orthopäde 1995;24:314–318.

61. Antti-Poika I, Josefson G, Kottinen Y, Lidgren L, Santavirta S, Sanzén L. Hip arthroplasty infection. Acta Orthop Scand 1990;61:163–169.

Index